THE NEWEST DIABETIC COOKBOOK FOR BEGINNERS

The Up-To-Date Guide To 2000-Days Of Nourishing Diabetic-Friendly Recipes For Type 2 Diabetes, Newly Diagnosed And Pre-Diabetes, With A 31-Day Meal Plan To Control Blood Sugar

Marcus Baron

Table of Contents

COPYRIGHT © 2023

CHAPTER ONE

Introduction to Diabetes and Cooking

Understanding Diabetes: A Beginner's Guide

Diabetes is a chronic medical condition that affects how your body turns food into energy. When you eat, your body breaks down food into glucose, a form of sugar, which enters your bloodstream. In response, your pancreas releases insulin, a hormone that helps transport glucose from your bloodstream into your cells, where it can be used for energy. However, in people with diabetes, this process is disrupted, leading to elevated blood sugar levels.

There are several types of diabetes, including type 1, type 2, gestational diabetes, and prediabetes. Type 1 diabetes is an autoimmune condition in which the immune system attacks and destroys the insulin-producing cells in the pancreas. It typically develops in childhood or adolescence and requires lifelong insulin therapy. Type 2 diabetes is the most common form and is characterized by insulin resistance, where the body's cells do not respond effectively to insulin. This type of diabetes is often associated with lifestyle factors such as obesity, poor diet, and lack of exercise. Gestational diabetes occurs during pregnancy and usually resolves after childbirth, but it increases the risk of developing type 2 diabetes later in life. Prediabetes is a condition in which blood sugar levels are higher than normal but not high enough to be diagnosed as diabetes. However, without intervention, prediabetes often progresses to type 2 diabetes.

Managing diabetes involves maintaining blood sugar levels within a target range to prevent complications such as heart disease, stroke, kidney failure, nerve damage, and vision loss. This typically requires a combination of medication, lifestyle changes, and monitoring blood sugar levels regularly.

Importance of Diet in Diabetes Management

Diet plays a crucial role in managing diabetes, as the foods you eat directly impact your blood sugar levels. A well-balanced diet can help stabilize blood sugar levels, control weight, and reduce the risk of complications associated with diabetes. Here are some key principles to consider when planning meals for diabetes management:

1. **Carbohydrate Control**: Carbohydrates have the most significant effect on blood sugar levels, so it's essential to monitor carbohydrate intake carefully. Choose complex carbohydrates such as whole grains, fruits, vegetables, and legumes, which are digested more slowly and cause a gradual rise in blood sugar levels. Limit refined carbohydrates and sugary foods, which can cause rapid spikes in blood sugar.

2. **Balanced Meals**: Aim for balanced meals that include a combination of carbohydrates, protein, and healthy fats.

Protein and fat can help slow down the absorption of carbohydrates, preventing sharp increases in blood sugar levels after meals. Include lean proteins such as poultry, fish, tofu, and beans, as well as healthy fats from sources like nuts, seeds, avocado, and olive oil.

3. **Portion Control**: Controlling portion sizes is crucial for managing blood sugar levels and preventing overeating, which can lead to weight gain. Use measuring cups, spoons, or visual cues to portion out foods accurately, and avoid super-sized servings at restaurants. Pay attention to serving sizes listed on food labels and try to stick to recommended portions.

4. **Fiber-Rich Foods**: Fiber helps regulate blood sugar levels by slowing down the absorption of carbohydrates and improving insulin sensitivity. Include plenty of fiber-rich foods such as fruits, vegetables, whole grains, and legumes in your diet. Aim for at least 25-30 grams of fiber per day for optimal health benefits.

5. **Healthy Cooking Methods**: Opt for healthy cooking methods such as baking, broiling, grilling, steaming, or sautéing with minimal added fats. Avoid frying or deep-frying foods, which can add excess calories and unhealthy fats. Use herbs, spices, and citrus juices to flavor dishes instead of salt or high-calorie sauces.

6. **Hydration**: Stay hydrated by drinking plenty of water throughout the day. Limit sugary beverages such as soda, fruit juice, and sweetened tea or coffee, which can cause spikes in blood sugar levels. Opt for water, herbal tea, or sparkling water with a splash of lemon or lime for flavor.

7. **Regular Meal Timing**: Establish a regular meal schedule with consistent timing for breakfast, lunch, dinner, and snacks. Spacing out meals evenly throughout the day can help prevent large fluctuations in blood sugar levels and maintain energy levels.

8. **Monitoring Blood Sugar**: Monitor your blood sugar levels regularly using a glucometer to track how food, physical activity, medication, and other factors affect your blood sugar levels. This information can help you make informed decisions about your diet and lifestyle to better manage diabetes.

9. **Individualized Approach**: Work with a registered dietitian or certified diabetes educator to develop a personalized meal plan that meets your specific dietary needs, preferences, and lifestyle. They can provide guidance on portion control, carbohydrate counting, meal timing, and food choices to help you achieve your diabetes management goals.

By following these dietary principles and adopting healthy eating habits, you can better control your blood sugar levels, improve overall health, and reduce the risk of complications associated with diabetes.

Getting Started in the Kitchen: Essential Tools and Techniques

Cooking at home can be a valuable tool for managing diabetes, as it allows you to have greater control over the ingredients and portion sizes of your meals. Whether you're a novice in the kitchen or an experienced home cook, having the right tools and mastering essential cooking techniques can make meal preparation more efficient and enjoyable. Here are some essential tools and techniques to help you get started:

Tools

1. **Cutting Board and Knife**: A sturdy cutting board and sharp knife are essential for preparing fruits, vegetables, and other ingredients. Choose a cutting board made of non-porous material such as plastic or wood, and select a high-quality chef's knife that feels comfortable in your hand.

2. **Measuring Cups and Spoons**: Accurate measurement is crucial for portion control and following recipes. Invest in a set of measuring cups and spoons for dry and liquid ingredients to ensure consistent results.

3. **Cookware**: Stock your kitchen with a variety of cookware, including pots, pans, and baking sheets, in different sizes and

materials. Non-stick pans are ideal for cooking with minimal added fats, while stainless steel or cast iron pans are suitable for searing and browning.

4. **Food Scale**: A digital food scale is helpful for measuring ingredients by weight, especially for precise portion control and following recipes that list ingredients in grams or ounces.

5. **Glucometer**: If you have diabetes, a glucometer is an essential tool for monitoring your blood sugar levels at home. Choose a glucometer that is easy to use, accurate, and compatible with your lifestyle and preferences.

6. **Slow Cooker or Instant Pot**: These kitchen appliances are convenient for preparing healthy meals with minimal effort. Slow cookers are great for making soups, stews, and braised dishes, while Instant Pots offer the versatility of pressure cooking, slow cooking, sautéing, and more.

7. **Blender or Food Processor**: Blenders and food processors are useful for pureeing soups, making smoothies, chopping vegetables, and creating sauces and dips. Look for a high-powered blender or food processor with multiple settings and attachments for versatility.

8. **Storage Containers**: Invest in a set of reusable storage containers for storing leftovers, prepped ingredients, and

homemade meals. Choose containers that are microwave-safe, dishwasher-safe, and stackable for easy storage and organization.

Techniques

1. **Knife Skills**: Learn basic knife skills such as chopping, slicing, dicing, and mincing to prepare ingredients efficiently and safely. Hold the knife with a firm grip and use a rocking motion to guide the blade through the food, keeping your fingers tucked away from the blade to prevent injuries.

2. **Sauteing and Stir-Frying**: Sauteing involves cooking food quickly in a small amount of oil or fat over medium to high heat, while stir-frying involves cooking food rapidly in a wok or skillet with constant stirring. Master these techniques for cooking vegetables, meats, and grains with minimal added fats and maximum flavor.

3. **Steaming**: Steaming is a gentle cooking method that preserves the natural flavors and nutrients of foods without added fats. Use a steamer basket or bamboo steamer to cook vegetables, fish, poultry, and dumplings until tender and cooked through.

4. **Roasting and Baking**: Roasting and baking are dry-heat cooking methods that produce crispy textures and caramelized flavors. Preheat your oven to the desired temperature, season the ingredients with herbs and spices,

and place them on a baking sheet or in a baking dish. Roast vegetables, meats, poultry, and seafood until golden brown and cooked to perfection.

5. **Grilling**: Grilling is a healthy cooking method that adds smoky flavor and charred marks to foods without added fats. Preheat your grill to medium-high heat, brush the grates with oil to prevent sticking, and place the ingredients directly on the grill. Grill meats, fish, vegetables, and fruits until charred and cooked through, flipping them halfway through cooking.

6. **Meal Planning and Prep**: Plan your meals and snacks ahead of time to save time and ensure balanced nutrition. Create a weekly meal plan, make a shopping list, and prep ingredients in advance by washing, chopping, and portioning them into containers. Store prepped ingredients in the refrigerator or freezer for quick and easy meal assembly throughout the week.

7. **Recipe Modification**: Adapt recipes to fit your dietary preferences, nutritional needs, and diabetes management goals. Swap ingredients for healthier alternatives, such as using whole grains instead of refined grains, reducing added sugars, and increasing fiber-rich foods. Experiment with herbs, spices, and flavorings to enhance the taste of dishes without adding extra salt or calories.

8. **Mindful Eating**: Practice mindful eating by paying attention to hunger and fullness cues, savoring each bite, and eating slowly without distractions. Focus on the sensory experience of food, including its appearance, aroma, texture, and taste, to enhance satisfaction and enjoyment of meals.

By mastering these essential tools and techniques, you can become more confident and proficient in the kitchen, making it easier to prepare delicious and nutritious meals that support your diabetes management goals.

This comprehensive guide provides an overview of diabetes, the importance of diet in diabetes management, and essential tools and techniques for cooking at home. Whether you're newly diagnosed with diabetes or looking to improve your culinary skills, incorporating these principles into your daily routine can help you take control of your health and well-being.

CHAPTER TWO

Basics of Meal Planning for Diabetes

Introduction to Meal Planning for Beginners

Meal planning is a fundamental aspect of managing diabetes, as it allows you to make informed food choices that help regulate blood sugar levels and promote overall health. Whether you're new to diabetes or looking to improve your meal planning skills, understanding the basics can set you on the path to success. Here's an introduction to meal planning for beginners:

1. **Setting Goals**: Start by identifying your dietary goals and preferences. Consider factors such as blood sugar control, weight management, nutritional needs, taste preferences, cultural influences, and budget constraints. Setting realistic and achievable goals can help you stay motivated and focused on making positive changes to your diet.

2. **Understanding Carbohydrates**: Carbohydrates have the most significant impact on blood sugar levels, so it's essential to monitor your carbohydrate intake carefully. Choose complex carbohydrates such as whole grains, fruits, vegetables, and legumes, which are rich in fiber and digested more slowly, leading to gradual increases in blood sugar levels. Limit refined carbohydrates and sugary foods, which can cause rapid spikes in blood sugar.

3. **Balancing Macronutrients**: Aim for balanced meals that include a combination of carbohydrates, protein, and healthy fats. Protein and fat can help slow down the absorption of carbohydrates, preventing sharp increases in blood sugar levels after meals. Include lean proteins such as poultry, fish, tofu, and beans, as well as healthy fats from sources like nuts, seeds, avocado, and olive oil.

4. **Meal Timing**: Establish a regular meal schedule with consistent timing for breakfast, lunch, dinner, and snacks. Spacing out meals evenly throughout the day can help prevent large fluctuations in blood sugar levels and maintain energy levels. Aim to eat every 3-4 hours to keep blood sugar stable and avoid overeating.

5. **Portion Control**: Pay attention to portion sizes to prevent overeating and promote weight management. Use measuring cups, spoons, or visual cues to portion out foods accurately, and avoid super-sized servings at restaurants. Be mindful of serving sizes listed on food labels and aim to stick to recommended portions to control calorie and carbohydrate intake.

6. **Meal Variety**: Include a variety of foods from all food groups to ensure balanced nutrition and prevent dietary boredom. Experiment with different fruits, vegetables, whole grains, lean proteins, and healthy fats to add variety to your meals

and snacks. Try new recipes and cooking techniques to keep meals interesting and enjoyable.

7. **Hydration**: Stay hydrated by drinking plenty of water throughout the day. Limit sugary beverages such as soda, fruit juice, and sweetened tea or coffee, which can cause spikes in blood sugar levels. Opt for water, herbal tea, or sparkling water with a splash of lemon or lime for flavor.

8. **Planning Ahead**: Plan your meals and snacks ahead of time to save time and reduce stress during busy weekdays. Create a weekly meal plan, make a shopping list, and prep ingredients in advance by washing, chopping, and portioning them into containers. Having healthy options readily available can prevent impulsive food choices and help you stay on track with your diabetes management goals.

By following these meal planning basics for beginners, you can take control of your diet and effectively manage your diabetes while enjoying delicious and nutritious meals.

Balancing Macronutrients: Carbohydrates, Proteins, and Fats

Balancing macronutrients—carbohydrates, proteins, and fats—is crucial for managing blood sugar levels, promoting satiety, and maintaining overall health. Each macronutrient plays a unique role in your diet, and finding the right balance can help you achieve optimal nutrition and diabetes management. Here's a closer look at each macronutrient and how to balance them in your meals:

1. **Carbohydrates**: Carbohydrates are the body's primary source of energy and have the most significant impact on blood sugar levels. When consumed, carbohydrates are broken down into glucose, which enters the bloodstream and raises blood sugar levels. For people with diabetes, monitoring carbohydrate intake is essential for controlling blood sugar levels and preventing spikes and crashes.

   - **Types of Carbohydrates**: Carbohydrates can be categorized as simple or complex based on their chemical structure and how quickly they are digested and absorbed by the body. Simple carbohydrates include sugars such as sucrose, fructose, and lactose, found in foods like fruits, honey, and dairy products. Complex carbohydrates include starches and fiber found in whole grains, legumes, fruits, and vegetables.

   - **Fiber**: Fiber is a type of carbohydrate that is not fully digested by the body and has many health benefits, including promoting digestive health, regulating blood sugar levels, and reducing the risk of heart disease. Aim to include plenty of fiber-rich foods such as fruits, vegetables, whole grains, and legumes in your diet.

- **Carbohydrate Counting**: Carbohydrate counting is a meal planning method that involves monitoring the grams of carbohydrates in foods and adjusting insulin doses or medication accordingly. Work with a registered dietitian or certified diabetes educator to learn how to count carbohydrates and incorporate this technique into your meal planning routine.

2. **Proteins**: Proteins are essential for building and repairing tissues, supporting immune function, and maintaining muscle mass. Unlike carbohydrates, proteins have minimal impact on blood sugar levels and can help stabilize blood sugar by slowing down the absorption of carbohydrates. Include lean sources of protein such as poultry, fish, tofu, eggs, and legumes in your meals to promote satiety and balance blood sugar levels.

   - **Portion Sizes**: Aim to include a palm-sized portion of protein in each meal, along with a balance of carbohydrates, vegetables, and healthy fats. Be mindful of portion sizes to prevent overconsumption of protein, which can contribute to excess calorie intake and weight gain.

   - **Plant-Based Proteins**: If you follow a vegetarian or vegan diet, incorporate plant-based sources of protein such as beans, lentils, tofu, tempeh, nuts, and seeds into your meals to meet your protein needs. These foods are also rich in fiber, vitamins, minerals, and phytonutrients that support overall health and well-being.

3. **Fats**: Fats are an essential macronutrient that provides energy, supports cell growth, protects organs, and helps absorb fat-soluble vitamins. While fats have a higher calorie density compared to carbohydrates and protein, they play a vital role in a balanced diet when consumed in moderation. Focus on incorporating healthy fats such as monounsaturated and polyunsaturated fats into your meals while limiting saturated and trans fats.

   - **Healthy Fats**: Sources of healthy fats include avocados, nuts, seeds, olive oil, fatty fish (such as salmon, mackerel, and sardines), and flaxseeds. These fats are associated with numerous health benefits, including reducing inflammation, improving heart health, and supporting brain function.

   - **Portion Control**: Be mindful of portion sizes when including fats in your meals, as they are calorie-dense and can contribute to weight gain if consumed in excess. Use measuring spoons or visual cues to portion out fats such as oils, nut butters, and avocado to avoid overconsumption.

- **Limiting Unhealthy Fats**: Limit your intake of saturated fats and trans fats, which are found in foods such as red meat, full-fat dairy products, fried foods, processed snacks, and baked goods. These fats can raise cholesterol levels and increase the risk of heart disease when consumed in excess.

Balancing carbohydrates, proteins, and fats in your meals can help regulate blood sugar levels, promote satiety, and support overall health. Experiment with different food combinations, portion sizes, and meal timing to find the right balance that works for you and your diabetes management goals.

Portion Control and Serving Sizes

Portion control is a critical aspect of managing diabetes and promoting healthy eating habits. By understanding appropriate serving sizes and practicing portion control, you can better regulate blood sugar levels, manage weight, and prevent overeating. Here's a closer look at portion control and serving sizes:

1. **Understanding Serving Sizes**: A serving size is a standardized amount of food or drink used as a reference for nutritional information on food labels and dietary guidelines. Serving sizes can vary depending on the type of food and the recommendations of health organizations. It's essential to

familiarize yourself with serving sizes to make informed food choices and monitor your calorie and nutrient intake.

- **Food Labels**: Pay attention to serving sizes listed on food labels to determine how many servings are in a package and the corresponding nutritional content per serving. Use this information to track your intake of calories, carbohydrates, protein, fat, fiber, sodium, and other nutrients.

- **Visual Cues**: Use visual cues to estimate portion sizes when dining out or preparing meals at home. For example, a serving of protein (such as meat, fish, or tofu) is about the size of a deck of cards, a serving of carbohydrates (such as rice or pasta) is about the size of a tennis ball, and a serving of fat (such as oil or butter) is about the size of a thumb.

- **Measuring Tools**: Use measuring cups, spoons, or a food scale to accurately portion out foods and beverages, especially when cooking or baking. Measuring tools can help you control portion sizes and prevent overeating, which can lead to weight gain and blood sugar spikes.

2. **Plate Method**: The plate method is a simple and practical tool for portion control that can help you balance your meals and control blood sugar levels. Divide your plate into

sections and fill half with non-starchy vegetables, a quarter with lean protein, and a quarter with whole grains or starchy vegetables. This method ensures a balanced intake of carbohydrates, protein, and fiber-rich foods while controlling portion sizes.

- **Non-Starchy Vegetables**: Fill half of your plate with non-starchy vegetables such as leafy greens, broccoli, cauliflower, bell peppers, carrots, cucumbers, tomatoes, and zucchini. These vegetables are low in calories and carbohydrates but rich in vitamins, minerals, and fiber that support overall health and blood sugar control.

- **Lean Protein**: Fill a quarter of your plate with lean sources of protein such as poultry, fish, tofu, eggs, or legumes. Protein helps regulate blood sugar levels, promote satiety, and support muscle growth and repair. Choose lean cuts of meat, remove visible fat, and opt for cooking methods that don't add extra fat or calories.

- **Whole Grains or Starchy Vegetables**: Fill the remaining quarter of your plate with whole grains or starchy vegetables such as brown rice, quinoa, barley, whole wheat pasta, sweet potatoes, or corn. These foods provide energy, fiber, and essential nutrients while helping you feel full and satisfied.

3. **Mindful Eating**: Practice mindful eating by paying attention to hunger and fullness cues, eating slowly, and savoring each bite. Avoid distractions such as television, computers, or smartphones while eating, and focus on the sensory experience of food, including its appearance, aroma, texture, and taste. By tuning into your body's signals, you can prevent overeating and make more conscious food choices.

4. **Meal Planning**: Plan your meals and snacks ahead of time to prevent impulsive food choices and control portion sizes. Create a weekly meal plan, make a shopping list, and prep ingredients in advance by washing, chopping, and portioning them into containers. Having healthy options readily available can help you stick to appropriate portion sizes and maintain consistency with your diabetes management goals.

5. **Practicing Moderation**: Enjoy your favorite foods in moderation while being mindful of portion sizes and overall dietary balance. Allow yourself occasional treats or indulgences, but aim to balance them with healthier choices and portion control throughout the day. Remember that no single food or meal will make or break your diabetes management, so focus on long-term consistency and balance.

By practicing portion control and paying attention to serving sizes, you can better manage your blood sugar levels, promote weight management, and support overall health and well-being. Experiment with different portion control strategies and find what works best for you and your lifestyle to achieve your diabetes management goals.

CHAPTER THREE

Essential Kitchen Tools and Cooking Techniques

Must-Have Tools for Your Diabetic Kitchen

Equipping your kitchen with the right tools can make meal preparation easier, more efficient, and more enjoyable, especially when managing diabetes. Whether you're a novice cook or an experienced chef, having essential kitchen tools on hand can help you create delicious and nutritious meals that support your diabetes management goals. Here are some must-have tools for your diabetic kitchen:

1. **Cutting Board and Knife**: A sturdy cutting board and sharp knife are essential for chopping, slicing, and dicing fruits, vegetables, and other ingredients. Choose a cutting board made of non-porous material such as plastic or wood, and select a high-quality chef's knife that feels comfortable in your hand.

2. **Measuring Cups and Spoons**: Accurate measurement is crucial for portion control and following recipes. Invest in a set of measuring cups and spoons for dry and liquid ingredients to ensure consistent results.

3. **Cookware**: Stock your kitchen with a variety of cookware, including pots, pans, and baking sheets, in different sizes and

materials. Non-stick pans are ideal for cooking with minimal added fats, while stainless steel or cast iron pans are suitable for searing and browning.

4. **Food Scale**: A digital food scale is helpful for measuring ingredients by weight, especially for precise portion control and following recipes that list ingredients in grams or ounces.

5. **Glucometer**: If you have diabetes, a glucometer is an essential tool for monitoring your blood sugar levels at home. Choose a glucometer that is easy to use, accurate, and compatible with your lifestyle and preferences.

6. **Slow Cooker or Instant Pot**: These kitchen appliances are convenient for preparing healthy meals with minimal effort. Slow cookers are great for making soups, stews, and braised dishes, while Instant Pots offer the versatility of pressure cooking, slow cooking, sautéing, and more.

7. **Blender or Food Processor**: Blenders and food processors are useful for pureeing soups, making smoothies, chopping vegetables, and creating sauces and dips. Look for a high-powered blender or food processor with multiple settings and attachments for versatility.

8. **Storage Containers**: Invest in a set of reusable storage containers for storing leftovers, prepped ingredients, and

homemade meals. Choose containers that are microwave-safe, dishwasher-safe, and stackable for easy storage and organization.

Having these essential kitchen tools on hand can streamline meal preparation, enhance culinary creativity, and support your efforts to manage diabetes through healthy eating habits.

Basic Cooking Techniques for Beginners

Mastering basic cooking techniques is essential for creating delicious and nutritious meals at home, especially when managing diabetes. Whether you're a beginner cook or looking to refine your skills, learning fundamental cooking techniques can help you become more confident and proficient in the kitchen. Here are some basic cooking techniques for beginners:

1. **Sauteing**: Sauteing involves cooking food quickly in a small amount of oil or fat over medium to high heat. It's a versatile cooking technique that works well for vegetables, meats, poultry, seafood, and tofu. To sauté, heat a skillet or frying pan over medium-high heat, add a small amount of oil or fat, and cook the ingredients until they are tender and lightly browned, stirring frequently.

2. **Roasting**: Roasting is a dry-heat cooking method that uses high heat to cook food evenly and develop rich flavors and textures. It's commonly used for vegetables, meats, poultry, seafood, and tofu. To roast, preheat your oven to the

desired temperature, season the ingredients with herbs and spices, and spread them out in a single layer on a baking sheet or roasting pan. Roast the ingredients until they are tender and golden brown, flipping them halfway through cooking for even browning.

3. **Steaming**: Steaming is a gentle cooking method that preserves the natural flavors and nutrients of foods without added fats. It's ideal for vegetables, fish, poultry, and dumplings. To steam, bring a small amount of water to a boil in a pot or steamer basket, add the ingredients to the steamer basket, cover with a lid, and cook until the ingredients are tender and cooked through.

4. **Boiling**: Boiling is a moist-heat cooking method that involves cooking food in a liquid at or near its boiling point. It's commonly used for pasta, grains, legumes, eggs, and vegetables. To boil, bring a pot of water to a rolling boil, add the ingredients, and cook until they are tender and cooked through. Drain the ingredients and season as desired.

5. **Grilling**: Grilling is a healthy cooking method that adds smoky flavor and charred marks to foods without added fats. It's great for meats, poultry, seafood, vegetables, and fruits. To grill, preheat your grill to medium-high heat, brush the grates with oil to prevent sticking, and place the ingredients directly on the grill. Grill the ingredients until they are

charred and cooked through, flipping them halfway through cooking for even grill marks.

6. **Baking**: Baking is a dry-heat cooking method that uses oven heat to cook food evenly and develop crispy textures and caramelized flavors. It's commonly used for bread, pastries, cookies, cakes, casseroles, and roasted vegetables. To bake, preheat your oven to the desired temperature, place the ingredients in a baking dish or on a baking sheet, and bake until they are golden brown and cooked through.

7. **Stir-Frying**: Stir-frying is a quick and efficient cooking method that involves cooking food rapidly in a hot pan or wok with constant stirring. It's commonly used for vegetables, meats, poultry, seafood, tofu, and noodles. To stir-fry, heat a wok or skillet over high heat, add a small amount of oil, and cook the ingredients until they are tender and lightly browned, stirring constantly to prevent sticking and ensure even cooking.

By mastering these basic cooking techniques, you can create a wide range of delicious and nutritious meals at home while managing diabetes through healthy eating habits.

Tips for Meal Preparation and Organization

Meal preparation and organization are key components of successful diabetes management, as they can help you save time, reduce stress, and make healthier food choices throughout the week. Whether you're planning meals for yourself or your family, incorporating these tips can streamline the meal preparation process and support your efforts to eat well and stay on track with your diabetes management goals:

1. **Plan Ahead**: Take time to plan your meals and snacks for the week ahead. Create a weekly meal plan that includes a variety of foods from all food groups, taking into account your dietary preferences, nutritional needs, and diabetes management goals. Use a meal planning template or app to organize your meals and make a shopping list of ingredients you'll need.

2. **Batch Cooking**: Consider batch cooking large quantities of staple ingredients such as grains, proteins, and vegetables that can be used in multiple meals throughout the week. Cook grains like rice, quinoa, or pasta in bulk and store them in portioned containers in the refrigerator or freezer. Similarly, cook batches of lean proteins such as chicken, tofu, or beans and divide them into individual servings for easy meal assembly.

3. **Prep Ingredients in Advance**: Wash, chop, and portion out ingredients in advance to save time and streamline meal preparation. Prep fruits and vegetables for snacks and salads, marinate meats and tofu for quick stir-fries or grilling,

and portion out ingredients for recipes to make cooking more efficient during the week.

4. **Use Time-Saving Appliances**: Take advantage of time-saving appliances such as slow cookers, Instant Pots, and food processors to simplify meal preparation. Slow cookers are great for making soups, stews, and braised dishes with minimal hands-on time, while Instant Pots offer the versatility of pressure cooking, slow cooking, sautéing, and more. Food processors are useful for chopping, shredding, and pureeing ingredients quickly and efficiently.

5. **Portion Control**: Be mindful of portion sizes when preparing and serving meals to prevent overeating and support weight management. Use measuring cups, spoons, or visual cues to portion out foods accurately, and avoid super-sized servings at restaurants. Pay attention to serving sizes listed on food labels and aim to stick to recommended portions to control calorie and carbohydrate intake.

6. **Organize Your Kitchen**: Keep your kitchen organized and well-stocked with essential ingredients and tools to make meal preparation more efficient. Store frequently used items such as cooking oils, spices, and pantry staples in easy-to-reach locations, and declutter countertops to create a clean and functional workspace. Invest in storage containers,

labels, and shelf organizers to keep ingredients organized and accessible.

7. **Schedule Meal Prep Time**: Set aside dedicated time each week for meal prep and cooking. Choose a day when you have the most time and energy to devote to meal preparation, such as a weekend day or a quiet evening during the week. Use this time to plan meals, shop for groceries, prep ingredients, and cook meals in advance to save time during busy weekdays.

8. **Pack Meals and Snacks**: Pack meals and snacks in portable containers or bento boxes to take with you on the go. Prepare grab-and-go options such as pre-portioned salads, vegetable sticks with hummus, yogurt parfaits, and trail mix for quick and convenient eating during work, school, or travel. Having healthy options readily available can prevent impulsive food choices and help you stay on track with your diabetes management goals.

By incorporating these tips for meal preparation and organization into your routine, you can save time, reduce stress, and make healthier food choices that support your diabetes management goals. Experiment with different strategies to find what works best for you and your lifestyle, and enjoy the benefits of a well-planned and organized kitchen.

CHAPTER FOUR

Quick and Easy Breakfasts

Simple Breakfast Ideas for Busy Mornings

Mornings can be hectic, but starting your day with a nutritious breakfast sets a positive tone for the rest of the day, especially when managing diabetes. Here are some simple breakfast ideas for busy mornings:

1. **Overnight Oats**: Prepare a batch of overnight oats the night before by combining rolled oats with milk (dairy or plant-based), yogurt, chia seeds, and your choice of sweetener (such as honey or maple syrup) in a jar or container. Refrigerate overnight, and in the morning, top with fresh fruit, nuts, seeds, or nut butter for added flavor and texture.

2. **Smoothie**: Blend together a smoothie using your favorite fruits, vegetables, protein powder, and liquid base (such as water, milk, or yogurt). Customize your smoothie with ingredients like spinach, kale, banana, berries, avocado, Greek yogurt, and almond milk. Pour into a travel cup for an on-the-go breakfast option.

3. **Whole Grain Toast**: Toast a slice of whole grain bread and top it with mashed avocado, sliced tomato, and a sprinkle of everything bagel seasoning or a drizzle of olive oil.

Alternatively, spread nut butter on toast and top with sliced banana or strawberries for a quick and satisfying breakfast.

4. **Yogurt Parfait**: Layer Greek yogurt with fresh fruit, granola, and nuts in a glass or jar to create a delicious and nutritious parfait. Experiment with different fruit combinations such as berries, mango, pineapple, or peaches, and choose a granola with minimal added sugars and whole grains for added crunch.

5. **Egg Muffins**: Make a batch of egg muffins ahead of time by whisking together eggs, vegetables, cheese, and herbs in a muffin tin. Bake until set and golden brown, then store in the refrigerator or freezer for a convenient grab-and-go breakfast option. Reheat in the microwave for a quick and protein-packed meal.

6. **Chia Pudding**: Mix chia seeds with milk (dairy or plant-based), sweetener, and flavorings such as vanilla extract or cocoa powder in a jar or container. Refrigerate for at least 2 hours or overnight until thickened, then top with fresh fruit, nuts, or coconut flakes before serving.

7. **Peanut Butter Banana Wrap**: Spread peanut butter or almond butter on a whole grain tortilla, then top with sliced banana and a sprinkle of cinnamon. Roll up the tortilla and enjoy it as a portable and satisfying breakfast option that

provides a balance of carbohydrates, protein, and healthy fats.

8. **Cottage Cheese Bowl**: Mix cottage cheese with chopped fruit, nuts, and a drizzle of honey or maple syrup for a quick and protein-rich breakfast option. Cottage cheese is high in protein and low in carbohydrates, making it a suitable choice for stabilizing blood sugar levels.

These simple breakfast ideas require minimal time and effort to prepare, making them perfect for busy mornings when you're short on time but still want to start your day with a nutritious meal.

Low-Carb Breakfast Options for Stable Blood Sugar

For individuals with diabetes, choosing low-carb breakfast options can help stabilize blood sugar levels and prevent spikes throughout the day. Here are some low-carb breakfast ideas to consider:

1. **Vegetable Omelette**: Whip up a vegetable omelette using eggs, spinach, bell peppers, onions, mushrooms, and tomatoes. Cook the vegetables in a non-stick skillet until tender, then pour beaten eggs over the vegetables and cook until set. Fold the omelette in half and serve with a side of avocado or salsa for added flavor.

2. **Greek Yogurt with Nuts and Seeds**: Enjoy a serving of Greek yogurt topped with chopped nuts (such as almonds, walnuts, or pecans), seeds (such as chia seeds or flaxseeds), and a drizzle of sugar-free syrup or honey. Greek yogurt is high in protein and low in carbohydrates, making it an excellent choice for stabilizing blood sugar levels.

3. **Baked Avocado Eggs**: Cut an avocado in half and remove the pit, then scoop out a small portion of the flesh to create a well. Crack an egg into each avocado half, season with salt, pepper, and your favorite herbs, then bake in the oven until the eggs are set. Serve with a side of mixed greens for a low-carb and nutrient-rich breakfast option.

4. **Chia Seed Pudding**: Make chia seed pudding using chia seeds, unsweetened almond milk, vanilla extract, and a sugar-free sweetener such as stevia or monk fruit. Refrigerate for at least 2 hours or overnight until thickened, then top with sliced strawberries, blueberries, or raspberries for added flavor and texture.

5. **Smoked Salmon Roll-Ups**: Spread cream cheese on slices of smoked salmon, then top with cucumber slices, avocado, and a sprinkle of everything bagel seasoning. Roll up the salmon slices and secure them with toothpicks for a low-carb and protein-packed breakfast option.

6. **Coconut Flour Pancakes**: Make pancakes using coconut flour, eggs, unsweetened almond milk, and baking powder for a low-carb alternative to traditional pancakes. Serve with a dollop of Greek yogurt and fresh berries for added protein and fiber.

7. **Breakfast Salad**: Enjoy a breakfast salad made with mixed greens, cherry tomatoes, cucumber slices, hard-boiled eggs, and avocado. Drizzle with olive oil and balsamic vinegar for a light and refreshing meal that's packed with nutrients and low in carbohydrates.

8. **Sardines on Whole Grain Crackers**: Top whole grain crackers with canned sardines packed in water or olive oil, then garnish with sliced radishes, lemon zest, and fresh herbs. Sardines are rich in omega-3 fatty acids and protein, making them a nutritious and low-carb breakfast option.

These low-carb breakfast options are delicious, satisfying, and can help support stable blood sugar levels throughout the day, making them ideal choices for individuals with diabetes.

Breakfast Meal Prep Tips and Recipes

Meal prepping breakfast in advance can save time and simplify busy mornings, especially when managing diabetes. Here are some breakfast meal prep tips and recipes to try:

1. **Egg Muffins**: Preheat your oven to 350°F (175°C) and grease a muffin tin with cooking spray. In a large bowl, whisk together eggs, diced vegetables (such as bell peppers, onions, and spinach), shredded cheese, and cooked protein (such as diced ham or turkey sausage). Pour the egg mixture into the prepared muffin tin, filling each cup about three-quarters full. Bake for 20-25 minutes or until the egg muffins are set and lightly golden brown. Let cool before storing in an airtight container in the refrigerator for up to 4 days.

2. **Overnight Chia Seed Pudding**: In a jar or container, combine chia seeds, unsweetened almond milk, vanilla extract, and a sugar-free sweetener such as stevia or monk fruit. Stir well to combine, then refrigerate overnight or for at least 2 hours until thickened. Top with sliced strawberries, blueberries, or raspberries before serving. Store leftovers in the refrigerator for up to 3 days.

3. **Greek Yogurt Parfait Jars**: In individual jars or containers, layer Greek yogurt with mixed berries, granola, and chopped nuts. Repeat layers until the jars are filled, then seal with lids and store in the refrigerator for up to 3 days. Grab a jar on your way out the door for a quick and portable breakfast option.

4. **Low-Carb Breakfast Burritos**: Cook scrambled eggs with diced vegetables (such as bell peppers, onions, and

mushrooms) in a non-stick skillet until the eggs are set. Spoon the egg mixture onto whole grain tortillas, then top with shredded cheese and salsa. Roll up the tortillas and wrap them individually in foil for easy reheating. Store in the refrigerator or freezer, then microwave until heated through before serving.

5. **Homemade Granola Bars**: In a large bowl, combine rolled oats, nuts, seeds, dried fruit, and a drizzle of honey or maple syrup. Press the mixture into a lined baking dish and bake at 350°F (175°C) for 20-25 minutes or until golden brown. Let cool completely before cutting into bars. Store in an airtight container at room temperature for up to 1 week.

6. **Make-Ahead Smoothie Packs**: Prep individual smoothie packs by combining frozen fruit, leafy greens, protein powder, and any other desired add-ins (such as chia seeds or flaxseeds) in resealable plastic bags. Store the packs in the freezer, then simply dump the contents into a blender with liquid (such as water, milk, or yogurt) and blend until smooth.

7. **Low-Carb Breakfast Casserole**: In a greased baking dish, layer cooked sausage or bacon, diced vegetables (such as bell peppers, onions, and spinach), shredded cheese, and beaten eggs seasoned with salt and pepper. Bake at 375°F (190°C) for 25-30 minutes or until the eggs are set and the

top is lightly golden brown. Let cool before slicing into squares. Store leftovers in the refrigerator for up to 4 days.

8. **Peanut Butter Banana Overnight Oats**: In a jar or container, combine rolled oats, unsweetened almond milk, mashed banana, peanut butter, and a sprinkle of cinnamon. Stir well to combine, then refrigerate overnight or for at least 4 hours until thickened. Top with additional sliced banana and a drizzle of honey before serving. Store leftovers in the refrigerator for up to 3 days.

By meal prepping breakfast in advance, you can save time, reduce stress, and ensure you have nutritious and satisfying options on hand to start your day off right, even on the busiest mornings. Experiment with different recipes and ingredients to find breakfast options that work best for you and your diabetes management goals.

CHAPTER FIVE

Delicious and Nutritious Lunches

Healthy and Filling Lunch Ideas

Finding delicious and nutritious lunch options is essential for maintaining energy levels and supporting overall health, especially when managing diabetes. Here are some healthy and filling lunch ideas to enjoy:

1. **Quinoa Salad**: Prepare a quinoa salad by combining cooked quinoa with chopped vegetables (such as cucumber, bell peppers, cherry tomatoes, and red onion) and fresh herbs (such as parsley or cilantro). Toss with a lemon vinaigrette dressing made with olive oil, lemon juice, garlic, salt, and pepper for added flavor.

2. **Stir-Fry**: Whip up a stir-fry using your favorite vegetables (such as broccoli, carrots, snap peas, and mushrooms) and protein (such as chicken, tofu, or shrimp). Stir-fry the ingredients in a skillet with garlic, ginger, soy sauce, and sesame oil until tender and cooked through. Serve over brown rice or cauliflower rice for a satisfying meal.

3. **Mason Jar Salads**: Layer mason jars with your favorite salad ingredients, starting with dressing on the bottom, followed by hearty vegetables, proteins, grains, and leafy greens.

When ready to eat, shake the jar to distribute the dressing evenly and enjoy a portable and customizable salad option.

4. **Grilled Chicken Wrap**: Fill a whole grain wrap with grilled chicken breast, lettuce, tomato, cucumber, avocado, and hummus for a protein-packed and satisfying lunch option. Roll up the wrap and slice it in half for easy handling and enjoy it with a side of fresh fruit or raw veggies.

5. **Vegetable Soup**: Make a batch of vegetable soup using a variety of colorful vegetables (such as carrots, celery, onions, zucchini, and spinach) simmered in a flavorful broth. Add cooked beans, lentils, or whole grains for added protein and fiber, and season with herbs and spices to taste.

6. **Salmon Salad**: Flake cooked salmon fillets over a bed of mixed greens and top with sliced strawberries, avocado, toasted almonds, and crumbled feta cheese. Drizzle with balsamic vinaigrette dressing for a light and refreshing salad option that's rich in omega-3 fatty acids and protein.

7. **Turkey and Veggie Lettuce Wraps**: Fill large lettuce leaves with sliced turkey breast, hummus, shredded carrots, cucumber sticks, and sliced bell peppers for a low-carb and gluten-free lunch option. Roll up the lettuce wraps and secure them with toothpicks for easy handling and enjoy with a side of fruit or Greek yogurt.

8. **Bean and Veggie Burrito Bowl**: Assemble a burrito bowl with cooked brown rice or quinoa, black beans or pinto beans, roasted vegetables (such as sweet potatoes, bell peppers, and onions), salsa, guacamole, and a dollop of Greek yogurt or sour cream. Customize the toppings to suit your taste preferences and enjoy a hearty and nutritious lunch.

These healthy and filling lunch ideas are easy to prepare and perfect for enjoying at home, work, or on the go, making them ideal choices for individuals managing diabetes.

Vibrant Salad Creations for Lunchtime

Salads are a versatile and nutritious option for lunch, offering a variety of flavors, textures, and nutrients in one meal. Here are some vibrant salad creations to enjoy at lunchtime:

1. **Greek Salad**: Toss together chopped romaine lettuce, cherry tomatoes, cucumber slices, red onion, Kalamata olives, and crumbled feta cheese in a large bowl. Drizzle with a lemon-herb vinaigrette dressing made with olive oil, lemon juice, garlic, oregano, salt, and pepper for a refreshing and tangy salad option.

2. **Caprese Salad**: Arrange slices of fresh mozzarella cheese, ripe tomato, and basil leaves on a platter or individual plates. Drizzle with balsamic glaze or a mixture of balsamic vinegar and olive oil, and sprinkle with salt and pepper for a simple and elegant salad that celebrates classic Italian flavors.

3. **Taco Salad**: Create a taco salad with mixed greens, seasoned ground turkey or beef, black beans, corn, diced tomatoes, shredded cheese, and crushed tortilla chips. Top with salsa, avocado slices, and a dollop of Greek yogurt or sour cream for a Tex-Mex inspired salad that's both satisfying and flavorful.

4. **Asian-Inspired Salad**: Combine shredded cabbage, carrots, bell peppers, edamame, and sliced almonds in a large bowl. Toss with a sesame ginger dressing made with soy sauce, rice vinegar, sesame oil, ginger, garlic, and honey for a crunchy and vibrant salad option with Asian-inspired flavors.

5. **Mediterranean Salad**: Mix together cooked farro, chopped cucumber, cherry tomatoes, red onion, olives, and feta cheese in a large bowl. Drizzle with a lemon-oregano vinaigrette dressing made with olive oil, lemon juice, garlic, oregano, salt, and pepper for a hearty and flavorful salad that's reminiscent of Mediterranean cuisine.

6. **Kale Caesar Salad**: Massage kale leaves with lemon juice and olive oil to tenderize them, then toss with homemade Caesar dressing made with Greek yogurt, lemon juice, garlic, anchovy paste, Dijon mustard, and Parmesan cheese. Top with whole grain croutons and additional Parmesan cheese for a nutritious twist on a classic Caesar salad.

7. **Protein-Packed Cobb Salad**: Arrange chopped romaine lettuce on a platter or individual plates, then top with rows of cooked chicken breast, hard-boiled eggs, crispy bacon, avocado slices, cherry tomatoes, and crumbled blue cheese. Serve with a side of creamy ranch dressing for a satisfying and protein-packed salad option.

8. **Fruit and Nut Salad**: Combine mixed greens with sliced strawberries, blueberries, raspberries, kiwi, and mango in a large bowl. Sprinkle with toasted almonds, walnuts, or pecans, and drizzle with a honey-lime vinaigrette dressing made with lime juice, honey, and olive oil for a refreshing and vibrant salad option.

These vibrant salad creations are loaded with flavor, nutrients, and textures, making them perfect for enjoying at lunchtime as part of a balanced and healthy diet, especially for individuals managing diabetes.

Easy-to-Make Sandwiches and Wraps

Sandwiches and wraps are convenient and versatile options for lunch, offering endless possibilities for fillings and flavors. Here are some easy-to-make sandwiches and wraps to enjoy:

1. **Turkey and Avocado Sandwich**: Spread whole grain bread with mashed avocado, then layer on sliced turkey breast, lettuce, tomato, and red onion. Add a smear of Dijon mustard or mayonnaise for extra flavor, and enjoy a classic

and satisfying sandwich option that's rich in protein and healthy fats.

2. **Vegetarian Hummus Wrap**: Spread a whole grain wrap with hummus, then top with sliced cucumber, bell pepper strips, shredded carrots, mixed greens, and feta cheese. Roll up the wrap and slice it in half for a flavorful and plant-based lunch option that's packed with fiber and nutrients.

3. **Grilled Vegetable Panini**: Grill sliced vegetables (such as zucchini, eggplant, bell peppers, and red onion) until tender and lightly charred, then layer them on whole grain bread with melted mozzarella cheese and fresh basil leaves. Press the sandwich in a panini press or grill pan until golden brown and crispy for a delicious and satisfying lunch option.

4. **Tuna Salad Lettuce Wraps**: Mix canned tuna with Greek yogurt, diced celery, red onion, lemon juice, Dijon mustard, salt, and pepper to taste. Spoon the tuna salad onto large lettuce leaves, then top with sliced tomato and avocado. Roll up the lettuce wraps and secure them with toothpicks for a light and protein-rich lunch option.

5. **Egg Salad Sandwich**: Mash hard-boiled eggs with Greek yogurt, Dijon mustard, chopped celery, green onions, and fresh dill in a bowl. Spread the egg salad on whole grain bread and top with lettuce leaves and tomato slices for a

classic and satisfying sandwich option that's perfect for lunch.

6. **Caprese Wrap**: Layer whole grain tortillas with sliced mozzarella cheese, ripe tomato slices, fresh basil leaves, and a drizzle of balsamic glaze or reduction. Roll up the wraps and slice them in half for a flavorful and vegetarian-friendly lunch option that celebrates the flavors of Italy.

7. **Chicken Caesar Wrap**: Toss cooked chicken breast with Caesar dressing, chopped romaine lettuce, and grated Parmesan cheese in a bowl. Spoon the chicken mixture onto whole grain tortillas and roll them up tightly for a portable and protein-packed lunch option that's perfect for enjoying on the go.

8. **BLT Wrap**: Cook bacon until crispy, then layer it on whole grain tortillas with lettuce leaves, sliced tomato, and mashed avocado. Roll up the wraps and slice them in half for a classic and satisfying lunch option that's perfect for bacon lovers.

These easy-to-make sandwiches and wraps are versatile, customizable, and perfect for enjoying at lunchtime, whether you're at home, work, or on the go, making them ideal choices for individuals managing diabetes. Experiment with different fillings, breads, and condiments to create your favorite flavor combinations and enjoy a delicious and satisfying lunch.

CHAPTER SIX

Flavorful Dinners for Every Palate

One-Pot Meals for Effortless Dinners

One-pot meals are a lifesaver for busy weeknights, offering convenience, minimal cleanup, and plenty of flavor. Here are some delicious one-pot meal ideas to try:

1. **Chicken and Rice Casserole**: In a large oven-safe skillet or casserole dish, combine boneless, skinless chicken thighs, rice, diced vegetables (such as carrots, bell peppers, and peas), chicken broth, and seasonings (such as garlic powder, onion powder, and paprika). Cover and bake in the oven until the chicken is cooked through and the rice is tender for a comforting and hearty dinner option.

2. **Vegetarian Chili**: In a large pot or Dutch oven, sauté diced onions, bell peppers, and garlic until softened. Add canned diced tomatoes, kidney beans, black beans, corn, vegetable broth, and chili powder, cumin, and smoked paprika for seasoning. Simmer until the flavors meld together and the chili thickens, then serve with your favorite toppings such as shredded cheese, avocado, and cilantro.

3. **Beef and Vegetable Stew**: Brown stew beef cubes in a Dutch oven or large pot, then add diced onions, carrots, celery, potatoes, and garlic. Pour in beef broth, canned diced

tomatoes, and seasonings (such as thyme, rosemary, and bay leaves) for flavor. Simmer on the stove or in the oven until the beef is tender and the vegetables are cooked through for a comforting and nourishing stew.

4. **Pasta Primavera**: Cook your favorite pasta in a large pot of boiling salted water until al dente, then drain and set aside. In the same pot, sauté diced vegetables (such as bell peppers, zucchini, cherry tomatoes, and spinach) until tender. Add cooked pasta back to the pot along with a splash of pasta water, grated Parmesan cheese, and fresh herbs (such as basil and parsley) for a vibrant and flavorful pasta dish.

5. **Shrimp and Sausage Jambalaya**: In a large skillet or Dutch oven, cook sliced sausage until browned, then add diced onions, bell peppers, and celery. Stir in canned diced tomatoes, chicken broth, long-grain rice, Cajun seasoning, and cooked shrimp for a spicy and satisfying jambalaya. Simmer until the rice is cooked through and the flavors meld together for a taste of New Orleans cuisine.

6. **Lentil and Vegetable Curry**: Sauté diced onions, garlic, and ginger in a large pot until fragrant, then add diced vegetables (such as carrots, potatoes, and cauliflower) and red lentils. Pour in canned coconut milk, vegetable broth, and curry paste for flavor. Simmer until the lentils are tender and the

vegetables are cooked through, then serve over cooked rice for a warming and aromatic curry.

7. **Creamy Mushroom Risotto**: Sauté sliced mushrooms in a large skillet or Dutch oven until golden brown, then add diced onions and garlic. Stir in Arborio rice and cook until translucent, then gradually add chicken or vegetable broth, stirring constantly until absorbed. Finish with a splash of white wine, grated Parmesan cheese, and chopped fresh herbs (such as parsley and thyme) for a creamy and decadent risotto.

8. **Quinoa and Black Bean Skillet**: Cook quinoa in a large skillet with diced onions, bell peppers, and garlic until tender. Stir in canned black beans, canned diced tomatoes, corn kernels, and Mexican seasoning blend for flavor. Top with shredded cheese, avocado slices, and fresh cilantro for a protein-packed and nutritious skillet dinner.

These one-pot meals are easy to prepare, packed with flavor, and perfect for satisfying hungry appetites at dinnertime, making them ideal choices for individuals managing diabetes.

Sheet Pan Dinners: Minimal Prep, Maximum Flavor

Sheet pan dinners are a game-changer for busy weeknights, offering minimal prep and cleanup while delivering maximum flavor. Here are some delicious sheet pan dinner ideas to try:

1. **Balsamic Chicken and Vegetables**: Marinate boneless, skinless chicken breasts in a mixture of balsamic vinegar, olive oil, garlic, and Italian seasoning for at least 30 minutes. Arrange the chicken on a sheet pan with assorted vegetables (such as bell peppers, zucchini, and cherry tomatoes) and roast in the oven until the chicken is cooked through and the vegetables are tender for a flavorful and balanced meal.

2. **Salmon and Asparagus**: Place salmon fillets on a sheet pan lined with parchment paper, then surround them with trimmed asparagus spears. Drizzle the salmon and asparagus with olive oil, lemon juice, minced garlic, and dill, then season with salt and pepper. Roast in the oven until the salmon is flaky and the asparagus is tender for a simple and elegant dinner option.

3. **Sausage and Potato Bake**: Cut smoked sausage into slices and toss with diced potatoes, sliced bell peppers, onions, and garlic on a sheet pan. Drizzle with olive oil and season with paprika, thyme, salt, and pepper. Roast in the oven until

the sausage is browned and the potatoes are crispy for a hearty and satisfying dinner option.

4. **Teriyaki Chicken and Broccoli**: Arrange chicken thighs on a sheet pan with broccoli florets and sliced bell peppers. Brush the chicken and vegetables with teriyaki sauce and sprinkle with sesame seeds, then roast in the oven until the chicken is cooked through and the vegetables are tender for a flavorful and Asian-inspired dinner option.

5. **Pork Tenderloin and Brussels Sprouts**: Season pork tenderloin with a mixture of garlic powder, onion powder, paprika, and thyme, then place it on a sheet pan surrounded by halved Brussels sprouts. Drizzle with olive oil and balsamic vinegar, then roast in the oven until the pork is cooked through and the Brussels sprouts are caramelized for a savory and satisfying dinner option.

6. **Honey Mustard Chicken and Potatoes**: Whisk together honey, Dijon mustard, minced garlic, and olive oil in a bowl, then toss with chicken thighs and quartered potatoes on a sheet pan. Roast in the oven until the chicken is golden brown and cooked through and the potatoes are tender for a sweet and tangy dinner option.

7. **Mediterranean Veggie Bake**: Toss diced eggplant, zucchini, bell peppers, red onion, and cherry tomatoes with olive oil, minced garlic, dried oregano, and lemon zest on a sheet pan.

Roast in the oven until the vegetables are tender and caramelized, then serve with cooked couscous or quinoa for a flavorful and vegetarian-friendly dinner option.

8. **Shrimp Fajita Bake**: Arrange shrimp, sliced bell peppers, and onions on a sheet pan lined with parchment paper. Drizzle with olive oil and sprinkle with fajita seasoning, then roast in the oven until the shrimp are pink and cooked through and the vegetables are tender. Serve with warm tortillas, salsa, guacamole, and sour cream for a Tex-Mex inspired dinner option.

These sheet pan dinners are easy to prepare, require minimal cleanup, and offer a variety of flavors and ingredients to suit every palate, making them perfect for busy weeknights when time is limited but flavor is not.

Quick and Healthy Stir-Fries and Skillet Dishes

Stir-fries and skillet dishes are quick, versatile, and perfect for busy weeknights when time is limited. Here are some quick and healthy stir-fries and skillet dishes to try:

1. **Chicken and Vegetable Stir-Fry**: Heat a large skillet or wok over medium-high heat and add diced chicken breast. Cook until browned and cooked through, then remove from the skillet and set aside. In the same skillet, add diced vegetables (such as bell peppers, broccoli, carrots, and snap peas) and stir-fry until tender-crisp. Add the cooked chicken back to

the skillet along with a sauce made from soy sauce, garlic, ginger, and honey. Cook until heated through and serve over cooked brown rice or quinoa for a quick and nutritious stir-fry.

2. **Beef and Broccoli Skillet**: Sauté thinly sliced beef sirloin strips in a large skillet over medium-high heat until browned, then remove from the skillet and set aside. In the same skillet, add broccoli florets and diced onions and cook until tender-crisp. Return the cooked beef to the skillet and add a sauce made from soy sauce, garlic, ginger, and brown sugar. Cook until heated through and serve over cooked rice or noodles for a flavorful and satisfying skillet dish.

3. **Shrimp and Veggie Stir-Fry**: Heat a large skillet or wok over medium-high heat and add peeled and deveined shrimp. Cook until pink and opaque, then remove from the skillet and set aside. In the same skillet, add diced vegetables (such as bell peppers, zucchini, mushrooms, and snow peas) and stir-fry until tender-crisp. Return the cooked shrimp to the skillet along with a sauce made from soy sauce, garlic, ginger, and hoisin sauce. Cook until heated through and serve over cooked rice or noodles for a quick and healthy stir-fry.

4. **Tofu and Vegetable Stir-Fry**: Press firm tofu to remove excess moisture, then cut it into cubes. Heat a large skillet or

wok over medium-high heat and add the tofu cubes. Cook until browned and crispy on all sides, then remove from the skillet and set aside. In the same skillet, add diced vegetables (such as bell peppers, broccoli, carrots, and snap peas) and stir-fry until tender-crisp. Return the cooked tofu to the skillet along with a sauce made from soy sauce, garlic, ginger, and sesame oil. Cook until heated through and serve over cooked brown rice or quinoa for a vegetarian-friendly stir-fry.

5. **Pork and Vegetable Skillet**: Brown thinly sliced pork tenderloin in a large skillet over medium-high heat until cooked through, then remove from the skillet and set aside. In the same skillet, add diced vegetables (such as bell peppers, onions, carrots, and cabbage) and cook until tender-crisp. Return the cooked pork to the skillet and add a sauce made from soy sauce, garlic, ginger, and honey. Cook until heated through and serve over cooked rice or noodles for a flavorful and nutritious skillet dish.

6. **Sesame Ginger Beef Stir-Fry**: Marinate thinly sliced beef sirloin strips in a mixture of soy sauce, sesame oil, minced garlic, grated ginger, and brown sugar for at least 30 minutes. Heat a large skillet or wok over medium-high heat and add the marinated beef, reserving the marinade. Cook until browned and cooked through, then remove from the

skillet and set aside. In the same skillet, add diced vegetables (such as bell peppers, broccoli, carrots, and snow peas) and stir-fry until tender-crisp. Return the cooked beef to the skillet along with the reserved marinade. Cook until heated through and serve over cooked rice or noodles for a flavorful and aromatic stir-fry.

7. **Cashew Chicken Skillet**: Sauté diced chicken breast in a large skillet over medium-high heat until browned and cooked through, then remove from the skillet and set aside. In the same skillet, add diced bell peppers, onions, and garlic and cook until softened. Return the cooked chicken to the skillet and add a sauce made from soy sauce, hoisin sauce, minced ginger, and honey. Cook until heated through and stir in roasted cashews for added crunch. Serve over cooked rice or noodles for a quick and flavorful skillet dish.

8. **Vegetable and Tofu Pad Thai**: Cook rice noodles according to package instructions, then drain and set aside. Heat a large skillet or wok over medium-high heat and add diced tofu. Cook until browned and crispy on all sides, then remove from the skillet and set aside. In the same skillet, add diced vegetables (such as bell peppers, bean sprouts, carrots, and green onions) and stir-fry until tender-crisp. Return the cooked tofu to the skillet along with the cooked rice noodles and a sauce made from tamarind paste, fish sauce, soy

sauce, garlic, and brown sugar. Cook until heated through and serve garnished with chopped peanuts, cilantro, and lime wedges for a flavorful and aromatic stir-fry.

These quick and healthy stir-fries and skillet dishes are easy to prepare, packed with flavor, and perfect for satisfying hungry appetites at dinnertime, making them ideal choices for individuals managing diabetes. Experiment with different proteins, vegetables, and sauces to create your favorite flavor combinations and enjoy delicious and nutritious dinners every night of the week.

CHAPTER SEVEN

Satisfying Snacks and Appetizers

Healthy Snacks to Curb Hunger Between Meals

Choosing healthy snacks can help manage hunger between meals and maintain stable blood sugar levels, especially for individuals managing diabetes. Here are some nutritious and satisfying snack ideas to try:

1. **Apple Slices with Peanut Butter**: Slice an apple and spread each slice with natural peanut butter for a satisfying combination of sweet and savory flavors. Apples are rich in fiber, while peanut butter provides protein and healthy fats to help keep you full between meals.

2. **Greek Yogurt with Berries**: Enjoy a serving of Greek yogurt topped with fresh berries such as strawberries, blueberries, or raspberries. Greek yogurt is high in protein and calcium, while berries are packed with antioxidants and fiber for a nutritious and refreshing snack option.

3. **Baby Carrots and Hummus**: Dip baby carrots in hummus for a crunchy and flavorful snack that's rich in fiber and protein. Hummus is made from chickpeas, which are high in protein and complex carbohydrates, while carrots provide vitamins, minerals, and antioxidants.

4. **Mixed Nuts**: Grab a handful of mixed nuts such as almonds, walnuts, and cashews for a satisfying and portable snack option. Nuts are rich in healthy fats, protein, and fiber, making them a nutritious choice to keep you feeling full and energized throughout the day.

5. **Hard-Boiled Eggs**: Enjoy a hard-boiled egg seasoned with a sprinkle of salt and pepper for a quick and protein-rich snack option. Eggs are a great source of high-quality protein and essential nutrients like vitamin D and choline, making them an excellent choice for managing hunger between meals.

6. **Cottage Cheese with Pineapple**: Serve cottage cheese with chunks of fresh pineapple for a creamy and tropical snack option. Cottage cheese is low in fat and high in protein, while pineapple provides natural sweetness and vitamin C for a refreshing and nutritious treat.

7. **Whole Grain Crackers with Cheese**: Pair whole grain crackers with sliced cheese for a satisfying and balanced snack option. Whole grain crackers are rich in fiber, while cheese provides protein and calcium to keep you feeling full and satisfied until your next meal.

8. **Edamame**: Enjoy a serving of steamed edamame pods sprinkled with sea salt for a protein-packed and satisfying snack option. Edamame is rich in plant-based protein, fiber,

and essential nutrients like folate and vitamin K, making it a nutritious choice for managing hunger between meals.

These healthy snacks are easy to prepare, delicious, and perfect for curbing hunger between meals, making them ideal choices for individuals managing diabetes.

Homemade Appetizers for Entertaining or Everyday Enjoyment

Homemade appetizers are perfect for entertaining guests or enjoying as a delicious snack any day of the week. Here are some flavorful and easy-to-make appetizer ideas to try:

1. **Caprese Skewers**: Thread cherry tomatoes, fresh mozzarella balls, and basil leaves onto small skewers or toothpicks. Drizzle with balsamic glaze and sprinkle with sea salt and freshly ground black pepper for a colorful and elegant appetizer option.

2. **Stuffed Mini Bell Peppers**: Cut mini bell peppers in half lengthwise and remove the seeds and membranes. Fill each pepper half with a mixture of cream cheese, chopped herbs (such as chives or parsley), and minced garlic. Bake until the peppers are tender and the filling is bubbly for a savory and satisfying appetizer option.

3. **Bruschetta with Tomato and Basil**: Top slices of toasted baguette with a mixture of diced tomatoes, minced garlic,

chopped fresh basil, extra virgin olive oil, balsamic vinegar, salt, and pepper. Serve immediately for a classic and flavorful appetizer that's perfect for any occasion.

4. **Spinach and Artichoke Dip**: Combine chopped spinach, marinated artichoke hearts, cream cheese, sour cream, mayonnaise, minced garlic, shredded mozzarella cheese, and grated Parmesan cheese in a baking dish. Bake until bubbly and golden brown, then serve with toasted bread or crackers for a creamy and indulgent appetizer option.

5. **Mini Quiches**: Line mini muffin tins with pastry dough and fill each cup with a mixture of beaten eggs, milk, shredded cheese, cooked diced vegetables (such as spinach, mushrooms, and bell peppers), and cooked crumbled bacon or sausage. Bake until set and golden brown for a delicious and portable appetizer option.

6. **Deviled Eggs**: Halve hard-boiled eggs lengthwise and remove the yolks. Mash the yolks with mayonnaise, Dijon mustard, minced shallot, and chopped fresh herbs (such as parsley or chives). Spoon the mixture back into the egg whites and sprinkle with paprika for a classic and crowd-pleasing appetizer option.

7. **Mushroom and Goat Cheese Crostini**: Sauté sliced mushrooms with minced garlic, thyme, salt, and pepper until tender and golden brown. Spread goat cheese onto toasted

baguette slices and top with the sautéed mushrooms. Garnish with chopped fresh parsley for a flavorful and elegant appetizer option.

8. **Baked Brie with Honey and Nuts**: Place a wheel of Brie cheese on a baking sheet and bake until softened and gooey. Drizzle with honey and sprinkle with chopped nuts (such as walnuts or almonds). Serve with sliced baguette or crackers for a decadent and irresistible appetizer option.

These homemade appetizers are easy to prepare, impressive, and perfect for entertaining guests or enjoying as a delicious snack any time, making them ideal choices for individuals managing diabetes.

Portable Snacks for On-the-Go Convenience

Portable snacks are convenient for busy lifestyles and provide a quick energy boost when you're on the go. Here are some portable snack ideas to try:

1. **Trail Mix**: Mix together nuts, seeds, dried fruit, and dark chocolate chips for a portable and energizing snack option. Trail mix is rich in healthy fats, protein, and fiber, making it a satisfying choice for on-the-go snacking.

2. **String Cheese and Grapes**: Pair string cheese with grapes for a convenient and portable snack option that combines protein and natural sweetness. String cheese is rich in

calcium and protein, while grapes provide hydration and vitamins.

3. **Nut Butter Packets with Whole Grain Crackers**: Spread individual packets of nut butter (such as almond or peanut butter) onto whole grain crackers for a portable and satisfying snack option. Nut butter is rich in healthy fats and protein, while whole grain crackers provide fiber and complex carbohydrates.

4. **Rice Cake with Avocado**: Top a rice cake with mashed avocado and a sprinkle of sea salt for a portable and nutritious snack option. Rice cakes are low in calories and fat, while avocado provides healthy fats, fiber, and vitamins.

5. **Greek Yogurt Parfait**: Layer Greek yogurt with mixed berries and granola in a portable container for a protein-packed and satisfying snack option. Greek yogurt is rich in protein and probiotics, while berries provide antioxidants and granola adds crunch and fiber.

6. **Hummus and Veggie Sticks**: Pack individual containers of hummus with sliced vegetables (such as carrot sticks, cucumber slices, and bell pepper strips) for a convenient and nutritious snack option. Hummus is made from chickpeas and is rich in protein and fiber, while vegetables provide vitamins, minerals, and hydration.

7. **Cottage Cheese with Pineapple Cups**: Pack individual containers of cottage cheese with chunks of fresh pineapple for a portable and refreshing snack option. Cottage cheese is low in fat and high in protein, while pineapple provides natural sweetness and vitamin C.

8. **Protein Bars**: Keep individually wrapped protein bars in your bag or car for a convenient and satisfying snack option when you're on the go. Look for protein bars that are low in added sugars and high in protein and fiber for sustained energy.

These portable snacks are convenient, nutritious, and perfect for on-the-go convenience, making them ideal choices for individuals managing diabetes. Pack them in your bag or lunchbox for a quick and satisfying snack option wherever your day takes you.

CHAPTER EIGHT

Wholesome Side Dishes to Complete Your Meals

Nutritious Vegetable Side Dishes

Vegetables are an essential part of a balanced diet, providing essential nutrients, fiber, and antioxidants. Here are some nutritious vegetable side dishes to complement your meals:

1. **Roasted Vegetables**: Toss assorted vegetables such as carrots, bell peppers, zucchini, and cauliflower with olive oil, garlic, and herbs (such as thyme or rosemary). Roast in the oven until tender and caramelized for a flavorful and nutritious side dish.

2. **Steamed Broccoli with Lemon Butter**: Steam broccoli florets until tender-crisp, then toss with melted butter, lemon zest, and a squeeze of lemon juice. Season with salt and pepper to taste for a simple and delicious vegetable side dish.

3. **Sautéed Spinach with Garlic**: Sauté fresh spinach leaves with minced garlic in olive oil until wilted. Season with salt, pepper, and a splash of lemon juice for a quick and nutritious vegetable side dish that pairs well with any main course.

4. **Grilled Asparagus with Parmesan**: Grill asparagus spears until tender and lightly charred, then sprinkle with grated

Parmesan cheese and a drizzle of balsamic glaze. Serve immediately for a flavorful and elegant vegetable side dish.

5. **Stuffed Bell Peppers**: Cut bell peppers in half lengthwise and remove the seeds and membranes. Fill each pepper half with a mixture of cooked quinoa, black beans, diced tomatoes, corn, and spices. Bake until the peppers are tender and the filling is heated through for a nutritious and colorful vegetable side dish.

6. **Glazed Carrots**: Cook baby carrots in a mixture of butter, honey, and orange juice until tender and glazed. Sprinkle with chopped fresh parsley for a sweet and savory vegetable side dish that's perfect for special occasions.

7. **Cauliflower Mash**: Steam cauliflower florets until tender, then mash with a potato masher or blend until smooth. Stir in a splash of milk, butter, and minced garlic for a creamy and low-carb alternative to mashed potatoes.

8. **Zucchini Noodles (Zoodles)**: Use a spiralizer to create noodles from zucchini, then sauté them in olive oil with garlic until tender. Season with salt, pepper, and freshly grated Parmesan cheese for a light and flavorful vegetable side dish.

These nutritious vegetable side dishes are easy to prepare, packed with flavor, and perfect for complementing a wide range of main courses, making them ideal choices for individuals managing diabetes.

Flavorful Grain and Legume Side Dishes

Grains and legumes are nutritious sources of carbohydrates, fiber, and protein, making them excellent options for satisfying and wholesome side dishes. Here are some flavorful grain and legume side dishes to try:

1. **Quinoa Salad**: Cook quinoa according to package instructions, then toss with diced vegetables (such as cucumber, bell peppers, cherry tomatoes, and red onion) and fresh herbs (such as parsley or cilantro). Dress with a lemon vinaigrette made with olive oil, lemon juice, garlic, salt, and pepper for a refreshing and nutritious grain side dish.

2. **Brown Rice Pilaf**: Sauté diced onions, garlic, and carrots in olive oil until softened, then add brown rice and cook until lightly toasted. Stir in vegetable or chicken broth and bring to a boil, then reduce the heat and simmer until the rice is tender and the liquid is absorbed. Fluff with a fork and stir in chopped fresh herbs (such as parsley or thyme) for a flavorful and wholesome grain side dish.

3. **Lentil Salad**: Cook lentils according to package instructions, then toss with diced vegetables (such as cucumber, bell

peppers, red onion, and cherry tomatoes) and crumbled feta cheese. Dress with a balsamic vinaigrette made with olive oil, balsamic vinegar, garlic, Dijon mustard, salt, and pepper for a protein-rich and satisfying legume side dish.

4. **Wild Rice Pilaf**: Cook wild rice according to package instructions, then toss with sautéed mushrooms, diced celery, dried cranberries, and chopped pecans. Season with salt, pepper, and a drizzle of olive oil for a hearty and flavorful grain side dish that's perfect for autumn or winter meals.

5. **Barley Risotto**: Cook pearl barley according to package instructions, then stir in sautéed onions, garlic, and mushrooms. Add vegetable or chicken broth gradually, stirring constantly, until the barley is creamy and tender. Stir in grated Parmesan cheese and chopped fresh parsley for a creamy and comforting grain side dish.

6. **Chickpea Salad**: Drain and rinse canned chickpeas, then toss with diced cucumbers, cherry tomatoes, red onion, and bell peppers. Dress with a lemon tahini dressing made with tahini, lemon juice, garlic, salt, and pepper for a flavorful and protein-packed legume side dish.

7. **Farro Salad**: Cook farro according to package instructions, then toss with roasted vegetables (such as butternut squash, Brussels sprouts, and cauliflower) and crumbled goat cheese.

Dress with a balsamic vinaigrette made with olive oil, balsamic vinegar, garlic, honey, salt, and pepper for a hearty and satisfying grain side dish.

8. **Black Bean and Corn Salad**: Drain and rinse canned black beans, then toss with cooked corn kernels, diced tomatoes, red onion, and cilantro. Dress with a lime vinaigrette made with olive oil, lime juice, garlic, cumin, salt, and pepper for a colorful and flavorful legume side dish.

These flavorful grain and legume side dishes are easy to prepare, versatile, and perfect for complementing a wide range of main courses, making them ideal choices for individuals managing diabetes.

Low-Carb Alternatives to Traditional Side Dishes

For individuals managing diabetes, incorporating low-carb alternatives to traditional side dishes can help manage blood sugar levels while still enjoying delicious and satisfying meals. Here are some low-carb alternatives to traditional side dishes to try:

1. **Cauliflower Rice**: Use a food processor or box grater to grate cauliflower into rice-sized pieces, then sauté in olive oil with minced garlic until tender. Season with salt, pepper, and chopped fresh herbs (such as parsley or cilantro) for a low-carb alternative to traditional rice.

2. **Zucchini Lasagna**: Use thinly sliced zucchini in place of lasagna noodles to create layers in a lasagna dish. Spread marinara sauce, ricotta cheese, shredded mozzarella cheese, and cooked ground turkey or beef between the layers of zucchini for a low-carb and gluten-free alternative to traditional lasagna.

3. **Spaghetti Squash Pasta**: Roast spaghetti squash halves in the oven until tender, then use a fork to scrape out the strands. Toss the spaghetti squash strands with marinara sauce, cooked vegetables, and grated Parmesan cheese for a low-carb alternative to traditional pasta.

4. **Mashed Cauliflower**: Steam cauliflower florets until tender, then mash with a potato masher or blend until smooth. Stir in a splash of heavy cream, butter, and minced garlic for a creamy and low-carb alternative to mashed potatoes.

5. **Eggplant Parmesan**: Use thinly sliced eggplant in place of breaded chicken or veal cutlets in a classic eggplant Parmesan dish. Layer the eggplant slices with marinara sauce, mozzarella cheese, and Parmesan cheese, then bake until bubbly and golden brown for a flavorful and low-carb alternative to traditional Parmesan dishes.

6. **Cucumber Noodle Salad**: Use a spiralizer or vegetable peeler to create noodles from cucumber, then toss with a light vinaigrette made with olive oil, vinegar, garlic, and herbs.

Add diced tomatoes, red onion, olives, and feta cheese for a refreshing and low-carb alternative to traditional pasta salad.

7. **Stuffed Portobello Mushrooms**: Remove the stems from portobello mushrooms and scrape out the gills. Fill the mushroom caps with a mixture of cooked spinach, ricotta cheese, minced garlic, and chopped fresh herbs. Bake until the mushrooms are tender and the filling is heated through for a flavorful and low-carb alternative to traditional stuffed dishes.

8. **Broccoli Cauliflower Gratin**: Steam broccoli and cauliflower florets until tender, then toss with a creamy cheese sauce made with heavy cream, cream cheese, shredded cheddar cheese, and seasonings. Bake until bubbly and golden brown for a decadent and low-carb alternative to traditional gratin dishes.

These low-carb alternatives to traditional side dishes are delicious, satisfying, and perfect for individuals managing diabetes who are looking to reduce their carbohydrate intake without sacrificing flavor or variety. Incorporate these dishes into your meal planning to enjoy wholesome and balanced meals that support your health and well-being.

CHAPTER NINE

Sweet Treats Without the Guilt

Sugar-Free Dessert Recipes for Indulgence Without the Spike

Enjoying sweet treats without worrying about blood sugar spikes is possible with these sugar-free dessert recipes. Here are some indulgent yet guilt-free options:

1. **Sugar-Free Chocolate Avocado Mousse**: Blend ripe avocados with unsweetened cocoa powder, a splash of almond milk, and a natural sugar substitute like stevia or erythritol until smooth and creamy. Chill in the refrigerator for a few hours before serving for a rich and decadent chocolate mousse without the added sugars.

2. **Low-Carb Cheesecake Bars**: Make a crust using almond flour, melted butter, and a natural sugar substitute, then press into the bottom of a baking dish. Beat cream cheese with eggs, vanilla extract, and lemon juice until smooth, then pour over the crust and bake until set. Chill before slicing into bars for a creamy and indulgent dessert option.

3. **Sugar-Free Peanut Butter Cookies**: Mix natural peanut butter with a sugar substitute like monk fruit sweetener, a beaten egg, and a splash of vanilla extract until well combined. Roll the dough into balls, place on a baking sheet,

and flatten with a fork. Bake until golden brown for a chewy and satisfying cookie without the added sugars.

4. **Stevia-Sweetened Lemon Bars**: Make a crust using almond flour, melted butter, and a natural sugar substitute, then press into the bottom of a baking dish. Whisk together eggs, fresh lemon juice, lemon zest, and stevia until smooth, then pour over the crust and bake until set. Chill before cutting into squares for a tangy and refreshing dessert option.

5. **Sugar-Free Chocolate Chip Blondies**: Mix almond flour with melted butter, a sugar substitute, vanilla extract, and sugar-free chocolate chips until well combined. Spread the batter into a baking dish and bake until golden brown and set. Let cool before slicing into squares for a chewy and irresistible blondie without the added sugars.

6. **No-Sugar-Added Berry Crisp**: Toss mixed berries with a natural sugar substitute, lemon juice, and a sprinkle of cinnamon, then place in a baking dish. In a separate bowl, mix almond flour, chopped nuts, melted butter, and a sugar substitute until crumbly, then sprinkle over the berries. Bake until bubbly and golden brown for a warm and comforting dessert option.

7. **Keto-Friendly Chocolate Pudding**: Heat almond milk in a saucepan until simmering, then whisk in unsweetened cocoa powder, a sugar substitute, and a pinch of salt until smooth

and thickened. Remove from heat and stir in vanilla extract and a knob of butter until melted. Chill in the refrigerator until set for a creamy and indulgent chocolate pudding without the added sugars.

8. **Sugar-Free Coconut Macaroons**: Mix shredded coconut with egg whites, vanilla extract, and a natural sugar substitute until well combined. Drop spoonfuls of the mixture onto a baking sheet lined with parchment paper and bake until golden brown and toasted. Let cool before enjoying these chewy and coconutty treats without the added sugars.

These sugar-free dessert recipes allow you to indulge in your sweet tooth without worrying about the negative effects of added sugars on your blood sugar levels, making them perfect for individuals managing diabetes.

Fruit-Based Desserts for Natural Sweetness

Harness the natural sweetness of fruits to create delicious and guilt-free desserts. Here are some fruit-based dessert ideas to satisfy your sweet cravings:

1. **Grilled Peaches with Honey and Cinnamon**: Halve fresh peaches and remove the pits, then brush with a mixture of honey and cinnamon. Grill until tender and caramelized, then serve with a dollop of Greek yogurt or a sprinkle of chopped nuts for a simple and satisfying dessert option.

2. **Mixed Berry Parfait**: Layer mixed berries such as strawberries, blueberries, and raspberries with Greek yogurt and a sprinkle of granola in individual glasses or jars. Repeat the layers until full, then garnish with a drizzle of honey or a sprig of mint for a refreshing and nutritious dessert option.

3. **Frozen Banana Pops**: Insert popsicle sticks into peeled bananas, then dip in melted dark chocolate and roll in chopped nuts, shredded coconut, or crushed graham crackers. Place on a baking sheet lined with parchment paper and freeze until firm for a fun and customizable dessert option.

4. **Watermelon Pizza**: Slice a watermelon into rounds and top with Greek yogurt or coconut yogurt, sliced strawberries, kiwi, and blueberries. Drizzle with honey and sprinkle with chopped mint or basil for a colorful and refreshing dessert option that's perfect for summer.

5. **Mixed Fruit Salad with Lime-Mint Dressing**: Combine diced fruits such as pineapple, mango, papaya, and kiwi in a bowl. Toss with a dressing made from fresh lime juice, honey, and chopped mint until well coated. Chill in the refrigerator before serving for a vibrant and flavorful dessert option.

6. **Baked Apples with Cinnamon**: Core fresh apples and place in a baking dish. Fill the center of each apple with a mixture of chopped nuts, raisins, cinnamon, and a drizzle of honey or

maple syrup. Bake until tender and caramelized for a warm and comforting dessert option.

7. **Frozen Yogurt Bark**: Spread Greek yogurt onto a baking sheet lined with parchment paper, then top with sliced fruits such as strawberries, kiwi, and blueberries. Drizzle with melted dark chocolate and sprinkle with chopped nuts or shredded coconut. Freeze until firm, then break into pieces for a refreshing and customizable dessert option.

8. **Mango Sorbet**: Blend frozen mango chunks with a splash of coconut milk and a squeeze of lime juice until smooth and creamy. Serve immediately for a tropical and refreshing dessert option that's naturally sweet and dairy-free.

These fruit-based dessert ideas allow you to indulge in delicious and satisfying treats while benefiting from the natural sweetness and nutritional value of fresh fruits, making them perfect for individuals managing diabetes.

Healthy Baking Tips and Tricks for Success

Baking can be both delicious and nutritious with these healthy baking tips and tricks:

1. **Use Whole Grain Flours**: Replace refined white flour with whole grain flours such as whole wheat flour, spelt flour, or almond flour for added fiber and nutrients in your baked goods.

2. **Reduce Added Sugars**: Cut back on the amount of sugar called for in recipes by using natural sugar substitutes such as stevia, monk fruit sweetener, or erythritol. You can also enhance sweetness with naturally sweet ingredients like ripe bananas, dates, or applesauce.

3. **Increase Protein Content**: Boost the protein content of your baked goods by adding ingredients like Greek yogurt, cottage cheese, or protein powder. This not only adds nutritional value but also helps keep you feeling full and satisfied.

4. **Incorporate Healthy Fats**: Replace unhealthy fats like butter or shortening with healthier options such as coconut oil, avocado oil, or olive oil. These fats provide heart-healthy benefits and can add richness and moisture to your baked goods.

5. **Add Fiber-Rich Ingredients**: Incorporate fiber-rich ingredients like ground flaxseed, chia seeds, or psyllium husk powder into your recipes to increase satiety and promote digestive health.

6. **Experiment with Alternative Sweeteners**: Explore alternative sweeteners such as maple syrup, honey, or molasses to add sweetness and flavor to your baked goods while reducing the overall sugar content.

7. **Include Nutrient-Dense Add-Ins**: Enhance the nutritional value of your baked goods by adding nutrient-dense ingredients like nuts, seeds, dried fruits, or shredded vegetables. These add-ins not only provide vitamins and minerals but also add texture and flavor to your creations.

8. **Practice Portion Control**: Enjoy your baked treats in moderation by practicing portion control. Cut larger desserts into smaller portions or make mini-sized versions to satisfy your sweet tooth without overindulging.

By incorporating these healthy baking tips and tricks into your culinary repertoire, you can create delicious and nutritious baked goods that support your health and well-being, making them perfect for individuals managing diabetes.

CHAPTER TEN

Dining Out with Diabetes

Strategies for Eating Out Healthily

Dining out can be enjoyable and stress-free even when managing diabetes with these strategies for eating out healthily:

1. **Plan Ahead**: Before heading to a restaurant, check the menu online if available. This allows you to review options and make informed choices ahead of time, reducing impulse decisions at the table.

2. **Choose Restaurants Wisely**: Opt for restaurants that offer a variety of healthy options, such as those with lighter fare, vegetarian or vegan choices, or customizable dishes. Ethnic cuisines like Mediterranean, Japanese, or Middle Eastern often have healthier options rich in vegetables, lean proteins, and whole grains.

3. **Control Portions**: Restaurant portions are often larger than necessary. Consider sharing an entrée with a dining companion or requesting a half-portion. Alternatively, ask for a to-go box upfront and portion out half of your meal before you start eating to avoid overeating.

4. **Ask for Modifications**: Don't hesitate to ask for modifications to suit your dietary needs. Requesting items

grilled instead of fried, sauces or dressings on the side, or substituting starchy sides with extra vegetables can help reduce excess calories and carbohydrates.

5. **Be Mindful of Hidden Sugars**: Beware of hidden sugars in sauces, dressings, marinades, and condiments. Opt for dishes with simple, transparent ingredient lists, and ask about sugar-free or low-sugar alternatives.

6. **Skip Empty Calories**: Avoid sugary drinks, alcoholic beverages, and high-calorie appetizers or desserts. Opt for water, unsweetened tea, or sparkling water with lemon or lime for a refreshing and calorie-free option.

7. **Balance Your Plate**: Aim for a balanced meal with a variety of food groups, including lean protein, non-starchy vegetables, whole grains, and healthy fats. This combination helps stabilize blood sugar levels and keeps you feeling satisfied longer.

8. **Practice Portion Control**: It's easy to overindulge when faced with a tempting menu. Practice portion control by ordering a starter salad or broth-based soup to start, which can help curb your appetite before the main course arrives.

By employing these strategies, you can navigate dining out with confidence and enjoy delicious meals while effectively managing your diabetes.

Making Smart Menu Choices at Restaurants

Making smart menu choices at restaurants is key to maintaining a balanced diet while managing diabetes. Here's how to make informed decisions:

1. **Start with Soup or Salad**: Begin your meal with a broth-based soup or a side salad with vinaigrette dressing. These options are typically lower in calories and can help control appetite before the main course.

2. **Focus on Lean Proteins**: Choose lean protein options such as grilled chicken, fish, tofu, or lean cuts of beef or pork. These protein sources are lower in saturated fat and can help stabilize blood sugar levels.

3. **Load Up on Vegetables**: Fill your plate with non-starchy vegetables like leafy greens, broccoli, cauliflower, bell peppers, and asparagus. These vegetables are high in fiber and nutrients but low in calories and carbohydrates.

4. **Watch Out for Hidden Sugars**: Be cautious of dishes that may contain hidden sugars, such as sweetened sauces, marinades, or glazes. Ask for sauces and dressings on the side or inquire about sugar-free options.

5. **Choose Whole Grains**: Opt for whole grain options when available, such as brown rice, quinoa, whole wheat pasta, or

barley. These complex carbohydrates provide more fiber and nutrients compared to refined grains.

6. **Customize Your Order**: Don't be afraid to customize your order to meet your dietary needs. Ask for substitutions or modifications to reduce added sugars, saturated fats, or excessive sodium.

7. **Portion Control**: Be mindful of portion sizes and avoid oversized servings. Consider sharing an entrée with a dining companion or ordering a half-portion to manage calorie and carbohydrate intake.

8. **Stay Hydrated**: Drink plenty of water throughout your meal to stay hydrated and help control appetite. Avoid sugary beverages and opt for calorie-free options like water, unsweetened tea, or sparkling water.

By making smart menu choices at restaurants, you can enjoy delicious meals while effectively managing your diabetes and promoting overall health.

Navigating Social Situations and Special Occasions

Navigating social situations and special occasions while managing diabetes requires planning and mindful choices. Here's how to stay on track:

1. **Communicate Your Needs**: Inform your friends, family, or dining companions about your dietary preferences and needs related to diabetes. This can help reduce misunderstandings and ensure that suitable options are available.

2. **Offer to Contribute**: If attending a gathering or potluck, offer to bring a dish that aligns with your dietary requirements. This ensures that there will be at least one option that you can enjoy without compromising your health goals.

3. **Scope Out the Menu in Advance**: If dining out at a restaurant, review the menu online beforehand to identify suitable options. Look for dishes that are lower in carbohydrates, saturated fats, and added sugars.

4. **Eat Before You Go**: If unsure about the food options available at an event, consider eating a balanced meal or snack beforehand. This can help prevent overindulging in high-calorie or high-carbohydrate foods.

5. **Practice Moderation**: Allow yourself to indulge occasionally but practice moderation and portion control. Enjoy small portions of your favorite treats without feeling guilty, and savor each bite mindfully.

6. **Stay Active**: Incorporate physical activity into your daily routine, especially on days when you anticipate consuming

more calories or carbohydrates than usual. This can help offset the effects of indulgent meals and keep blood sugar levels stable.

7. **Monitor Blood Sugar Levels**: Stay vigilant about monitoring your blood sugar levels, especially during social gatherings or special occasions. Keep necessary supplies on hand and be prepared to take action if levels become too high or too low.

8. **Focus on Enjoyment and Socializing**: Remember that social gatherings and special occasions are about more than just food. Focus on enjoying the company of friends and loved ones, engaging in meaningful conversations, and creating lasting memories.

By implementing these strategies, you can navigate social situations and special occasions with confidence while effectively managing your diabetes and prioritizing your health and well-being.

CHAPTER 11

DIET AND DIABETES

Mediterranean Diet:

Definition:

The Mediterranean diet is inspired by the traditional dietary patterns of countries bordering the Mediterranean Sea. It emphasizes whole, minimally processed foods such as fruits, vegetables, whole grains, nuts, seeds, legumes, fish, and olive oil. It limits red meat and sweets, while encouraging moderate consumption of dairy products, poultry, and eggs.

Ingredients:

- Fruits: Berries, apples, oranges, grapes, etc.

- Vegetables: Spinach, tomatoes, peppers, onions, etc.

- Whole Grains: Whole wheat bread, brown rice, quinoa, oats, etc.

- Nuts and Seeds: Almonds, walnuts, flaxseeds, chia seeds, etc.

- Legumes: Chickpeas, lentils, beans, etc.

- Fish and Seafood: Salmon, tuna, shrimp, etc.

- Olive Oil: Extra virgin olive oil for cooking and dressing.

- Herbs and Spices: Basil, oregano, garlic, cumin, etc.

Instructions/How to Prepare:

1. Base meals around plant-based foods like fruits, vegetables, whole grains, and legumes.

2. Use olive oil as the primary source of fat for cooking and dressing salads.

3. Incorporate fish and seafood into your diet regularly, aiming for at least two servings per week.

4. Enjoy moderate amounts of poultry, eggs, and dairy products, such as yogurt and cheese.

5. Limit red meat consumption to a few times per month.

6. Snack on nuts and seeds for a healthy source of fats and protein.

7. Flavor meals with herbs and spices instead of salt.

8. Drink plenty of water and enjoy a moderate amount of red wine if desired (optional).

DASH Diet (Dietary Approaches to Stop Hypertension):

Definition:

The DASH diet is specifically designed to help lower blood pressure and reduce the risk of hypertension. It emphasizes fruits, vegetables, whole grains, and lean proteins while limiting sodium, saturated fats, and sweets.

Ingredients:

- Fruits: Berries, bananas, apples, oranges, etc.

- Vegetables: Leafy greens, carrots, broccoli, bell peppers, etc.

- Whole Grains: Brown rice, whole wheat bread, quinoa, oats, barley, etc.

- Lean Proteins: Chicken breast, turkey, fish, tofu, beans, lentils, etc.

- Dairy: Low-fat or fat-free milk, yogurt, cheese, etc.

- Nuts and Seeds: Almonds, pistachios, sunflower seeds, etc.

- Healthy Fats: Olive oil, avocado, nuts, seeds, etc.

Instructions/How to Prepare:

1. Focus on incorporating plenty of fruits and vegetables into your meals and snacks.

2. Choose whole grains over refined grains whenever possible.

3. Opt for lean proteins such as poultry, fish, tofu, and legumes.

4. Limit high-fat dairy products and opt for low-fat or fat-free options.

5. Include nuts and seeds as snacks or in salads for added nutrients and healthy fats.

6. Use herbs, spices, and citrus juices to flavor foods instead of salt.

7. Avoid processed and high-sodium foods like canned soups, packaged snacks, and fast food.

8. Cook meals at home whenever possible to have better control over ingredients and portion sizes.

9. Aim to limit sweets and sugary beverages, opting for natural sweeteners like fruit when craving something sweet.

10. Stay hydrated by drinking plenty of water throughout the day.

Low-Carb Diet:

Definition:

A low-carb diet involves reducing carbohydrate intake while increasing the consumption of protein and healthy fats. This diet aims to control insulin levels, promote weight loss, and improve overall health by limiting foods high in carbohydrates such as bread, pasta, rice, and sugary snacks.

Ingredients:

- Protein Sources: Meat, poultry, fish, tofu, tempeh, eggs.

- Non-Starchy Vegetables: Leafy greens, broccoli, cauliflower, zucchini, bell peppers.

- Healthy Fats: Avocado, nuts, seeds, olive oil, coconut oil.

- Dairy: Cheese, Greek yogurt, cottage cheese (in moderation).

- Low-Carb Fruits: Berries, avocados, tomatoes, lemons, limes.

- Herbs and Spices: Basil, oregano, garlic, turmeric, cumin.

- Sweeteners (optional): Stevia, erythritol, monk fruit.

Instructions/How to Prepare:

1. Focus on whole, unprocessed foods.

2. Limit carbohydrate intake to around 20-50 grams per day, depending on individual needs and goals.

3. Include protein-rich foods in each meal to promote satiety and muscle maintenance.

4. Fill up on non-starchy vegetables to increase fiber intake and provide essential vitamins and minerals.

5. Incorporate healthy fats into your diet for energy and to keep you feeling full.

6. Be mindful of hidden carbs in sauces, condiments, and processed foods.

7. Drink plenty of water to stay hydrated and support overall health.

8. Experiment with low-carb recipes and meal prep to make adhering to the diet easier and more enjoyable.

Ketogenic Diet (Keto Diet):

Definition:

The ketogenic diet is a very low-carb, high-fat diet that forces the body to enter a state of ketosis, where it primarily burns fat for fuel instead of carbohydrates. This diet has been used for decades to treat epilepsy and has gained popularity for weight loss and improving metabolic health.

Ingredients:

- Healthy Fats: Avocado, coconut oil, olive oil, butter, ghee, fatty fish.

- Protein Sources: Meat, poultry, fish, eggs, tofu, tempeh.

- Non-Starchy Vegetables: Leafy greens, broccoli, cauliflower, zucchini, asparagus.

- Full-Fat Dairy: Cheese, heavy cream, Greek yogurt (in moderation).

- Nuts and Seeds: Macadamia nuts, almonds, chia seeds, flaxseeds.

- Low-Carb Fruits: Berries (in moderation), avocado.

- Herbs and Spices: Turmeric, ginger, cinnamon, garlic, thyme.

- Sweeteners (in moderation): Stevia, erythritol, monk fruit.

Instructions/How to Prepare:

1. Keep carbohydrate intake extremely low, typically below 20-50 grams per day to induce and maintain ketosis.

2. Consume moderate amounts of protein, as excessive protein intake can potentially hinder ketosis.

3. Base meals around healthy fats, such as avocados, olive oil, and fatty fish.

4. Incorporate non-starchy vegetables to provide essential nutrients and fiber while keeping carbohydrate intake low.

5. Be mindful of hidden carbs in foods and beverages, including sauces, dressings, and flavored beverages.

6. Stay hydrated by drinking plenty of water, as dehydration can occur more easily on a ketogenic diet.

7. Monitor ketone levels using urine strips, blood tests, or breath meters if desired, to ensure you are in ketosis.

8. Experiment with keto-friendly recipes and meal planning to maintain variety and enjoyment while following the diet.

Plant-Based Diet:

Definition:

A plant-based diet primarily consists of foods derived from plants, such as fruits, vegetables, grains, nuts, seeds, and legumes. It emphasizes whole, minimally processed foods while minimizing or eliminating animal products. The focus is on incorporating a variety of plant foods to promote health and well-being.

Ingredients:

- Fruits: Berries, apples, oranges, bananas, etc.

- Vegetables: Leafy greens, broccoli, carrots, bell peppers, etc.

- Whole Grains: Brown rice, quinoa, oats, barley, whole wheat bread, etc.

- Legumes: Chickpeas, lentils, black beans, kidney beans, etc.

- Nuts and Seeds: Almonds, walnuts, chia seeds, flaxseeds, pumpkin seeds, etc.

- Plant-Based Proteins: Tofu, tempeh, seitan, edamame, plant-based protein powders, etc.

- Healthy Fats: Avocado, olive oil, coconut oil, nuts, seeds, etc.

Instructions/How to Prepare:

1. Base meals around a variety of whole plant foods, including fruits, vegetables, whole grains, legumes, nuts, and seeds.

2. Incorporate a rainbow of colorful fruits and vegetables to ensure a diverse array of nutrients.

3. Include plant-based proteins such as tofu, tempeh, and legumes in meals to meet protein needs.

4. Choose whole grains over refined grains for added fiber and nutrients.

5. Experiment with different cooking methods, such as steaming, roasting, sautéing, and grilling, to enhance flavor and texture.

6. Use herbs, spices, and condiments to add flavor to dishes without relying on animal products.

7. Be mindful of nutrient needs, particularly vitamin B12, vitamin D, omega-3 fatty acids, iron, calcium, and zinc, and consider supplementation if necessary.

8. Stay hydrated by drinking plenty of water throughout the day.

9. Plan balanced meals and snacks to ensure adequate intake of essential nutrients.

10. Enjoy plant-based alternatives to dairy and meat products, such as plant-based milk, cheese, yogurt, and meat substitutes, if desired.

Vegan Diet:

Definition:

A vegan diet excludes all animal products, including meat, poultry, fish, dairy, eggs, and honey. It is based entirely on plant foods and emphasizes cruelty-free living and environmental sustainability.

Ingredients:

- Fruits: Berries, apples, oranges, mangoes, etc.

- Vegetables: Spinach, kale, tomatoes, onions, mushrooms, etc.

- Whole Grains: Quinoa, brown rice, barley, whole wheat pasta, etc.

- Legumes: Chickpeas, black beans, lentils, kidney beans, etc.

- Nuts and Seeds: Almonds, cashews, sunflower seeds, chia seeds, etc.

- Plant-Based Proteins: Tofu, tempeh, seitan, soy-based meat substitutes, etc.

- Healthy Fats: Avocado, olive oil, coconut oil, nuts, seeds, etc.

- Plant-Based Dairy Alternatives: Almond milk, coconut milk, soy milk, vegan cheese, vegan yogurt, etc.

Instructions/How to Prepare:

1. Build meals around plant foods, including fruits, vegetables, whole grains, legumes, nuts, and seeds.

2. Ensure adequate protein intake by including sources such as tofu, tempeh, legumes, and plant-based meat substitutes.

3. Use plant-based milk, cheese, and yogurt alternatives in place of dairy products.

4. Experiment with vegan cooking techniques and recipes to discover new flavors and textures.

5. Pay attention to nutrient needs, especially vitamin B12, vitamin D, omega-3 fatty acids, iron, calcium, and zinc, and consider supplementation if necessary.

6. Read labels carefully to avoid hidden animal ingredients in processed foods and beverages.

7. Be mindful of cross-contamination when preparing and consuming food to prevent unintentional consumption of animal products.

8. Explore vegan-friendly restaurants and eateries or plan ahead when dining out to ensure vegan options are available.

9. Connect with vegan communities and resources for support, recipe ideas, and lifestyle tips.

10. Embrace the ethical and environmental principles of veganism beyond diet by choosing cruelty-free and

sustainable products in other areas of life, such as clothing, cosmetics, and household items.

Vegetarian Diet:

Definition:

A vegetarian diet excludes meat, poultry, and seafood, but includes plant-based foods such as fruits, vegetables, grains, nuts, seeds, and dairy products. There are different variations of vegetarianism, including lacto-vegetarian (includes dairy but not eggs), ovo-vegetarian (includes eggs but not dairy), and lacto-ovo-vegetarian (includes both dairy and eggs).

Ingredients:

- Fruits: Berries, apples, oranges, bananas, etc.

- Vegetables: Leafy greens, broccoli, carrots, bell peppers, etc.

- Whole Grains: Brown rice, quinoa, oats, barley, whole wheat bread, etc.

- Legumes: Chickpeas, lentils, black beans, kidney beans, etc.

- Nuts and Seeds: Almonds, walnuts, chia seeds, flaxseeds, pumpkin seeds, etc.

- Dairy: Milk, yogurt, cheese, butter, etc. (depending on the type of vegetarianism)

- Plant-Based Proteins: Tofu, tempeh, seitan, edamame, etc.

- Healthy Fats: Avocado, olive oil, coconut oil, nuts, seeds, etc.

Instructions/How to Prepare:

1. Base meals around a variety of plant foods, including fruits, vegetables, whole grains, legumes, nuts, and seeds.

2. Incorporate plant-based proteins such as tofu, tempeh, legumes, nuts, and seeds into meals to meet protein needs.

3. Choose whole grains over refined grains for added fiber and nutrients.

4. Experiment with different cooking methods, such as steaming, roasting, sautéing, and grilling, to enhance flavor and texture.

5. Use herbs, spices, and condiments to add flavor to dishes without relying on meat.

6. Be mindful of nutrient needs, especially vitamin B12, vitamin D, omega-3 fatty acids, iron, calcium, and zinc, and consider supplementation if necessary.

7. Stay hydrated by drinking plenty of water throughout the day.

8. Plan balanced meals and snacks to ensure adequate intake of essential nutrients.

9. Explore vegetarian cooking techniques and recipes to discover new flavors and textures.

10.	Connect with vegetarian communities and resources for support, recipe ideas, and lifestyle tips.

Atkins Diet:

Definition:

The Atkins diet is a low-carbohydrate, high-fat diet designed for weight loss and improving overall health. It involves reducing carbohydrate intake while increasing the consumption of protein and healthy fats. The diet is divided into four phases: induction, balancing, fine-tuning, and maintenance.

Ingredients:

- Protein Sources: Meat, poultry, fish, eggs, tofu, tempeh, etc.

- Non-Starchy Vegetables: Leafy greens, broccoli, cauliflower, zucchini, bell peppers, etc.

- Healthy Fats: Avocado, olive oil, coconut oil, butter, ghee, fatty fish, etc.

- Full-Fat Dairy (in moderation): Cheese, Greek yogurt, heavy cream, etc.

- Nuts and Seeds (in moderation): Almonds, walnuts, chia seeds, flaxseeds, etc.

- Low-Carb Fruits (in moderation): Berries, avocados, tomatoes, etc.

- Herbs and Spices: Basil, oregano, garlic, turmeric, cumin, etc.

Instructions/How to Prepare:

1. Start with the induction phase, which restricts carbohydrate intake to 20-25 grams per day for two weeks to induce ketosis.

2. Base meals around protein-rich foods such as meat, poultry, fish, eggs, and tofu.

3. Include non-starchy vegetables to provide essential nutrients and fiber while keeping carbohydrate intake low.

4. Incorporate healthy fats into your diet for energy and to keep you feeling full.

5. Gradually increase carbohydrate intake during the balancing, fine-tuning, and maintenance phases while monitoring weight and overall health.

6. Be mindful of portion sizes and track carbohydrate intake to stay within the recommended limits for each phase.

7. Stay hydrated by drinking plenty of water throughout the day.

8. Experiment with low-carb recipes and meal planning to maintain variety and enjoyment while following the diet.

9. Consider working with a healthcare professional or registered dietitian to personalize the diet plan and ensure nutritional adequacy.

10.   Monitor progress and make adjustments as needed to achieve weight loss and health goals.

South Beach Diet:

Definition:

The South Beach Diet is a popular weight-loss program that emphasizes the consumption of lean protein, healthy fats, and low-glycemic carbohydrates. It's divided into three phases: Phase 1, which eliminates most carbs to jump-start weight loss; Phase 2, which reintroduces some carbs while continuing weight loss; and Phase 3, which focuses on maintaining weight loss with a balanced diet.

Ingredients:

- Lean Proteins: Chicken breast, turkey, fish, seafood, lean cuts of beef and pork.

- Healthy Fats: Olive oil, avocado, nuts, seeds, fatty fish like salmon and mackerel.

- Low-Glycemic Carbohydrates: Non-starchy vegetables (e.g., spinach, broccoli, cauliflower), whole grains (e.g., quinoa, barley), legumes (e.g., beans, lentils).

- Low-Fat Dairy: Greek yogurt, skim milk, low-fat cheese.

Instructions/How to Prepare:

1. Phase 1: Eliminate most carbohydrates, including fruits, grains, and starchy vegetables. Focus on lean proteins, non-starchy vegetables, and healthy fats. Drink plenty of water and avoid processed foods and added sugars.

2. Phase 2: Gradually reintroduce some carbohydrates, such as fruits and whole grains, while continuing to prioritize lean proteins and healthy fats. Monitor portion sizes and continue to avoid refined sugars and processed foods.

3. Phase 3: Transition to a balanced diet that includes a variety of foods from all food groups. Focus on portion control, mindful eating, and regular physical activity to maintain weight loss and overall health.

Paleo Diet:

Definition:

The Paleo diet, also known as the Paleolithic or caveman diet, is based on the presumed diet of ancient humans during the Paleolithic era. It emphasizes whole foods that would have been available to our hunter-gatherer ancestors, such as lean meats, fish, fruits, vegetables, nuts, and seeds, while excluding processed foods, grains, legumes, and dairy products.

Ingredients:

- Lean Meats: Beef, chicken, turkey, pork, lamb, etc.
- Fish and Seafood: Salmon, trout, shrimp, shellfish, etc.
- Fruits: Berries, apples, oranges, bananas, etc.
- Vegetables: Leafy greens, broccoli, carrots, peppers, onions, etc.
- Nuts and Seeds: Almonds, walnuts, cashews, sunflower seeds, etc.
- Healthy Fats: Avocado, olive oil, coconut oil, ghee.
- Herbs and Spices: Basil, oregano, garlic, turmeric, cinnamon, etc.

Instructions/How to Prepare:

1. Base meals around lean proteins, including meat, fish, and seafood.
2. Incorporate a variety of colorful fruits and vegetables for essential vitamins, minerals, and fiber.
3. Include nuts and seeds as snacks or to add texture and flavor to meals.

4. Use healthy fats like olive oil, avocado, and coconut oil for cooking and dressing.

5. Avoid processed foods, grains, legumes, dairy products, refined sugars, and artificial additives.

6. Experiment with cooking methods such as grilling, baking, and sautéing to enhance flavor and texture.

7. Stay hydrated by drinking plenty of water throughout the day.

8. Listen to your body's hunger and fullness cues and eat mindfully.

9. Be aware of portion sizes and adjust based on individual energy needs and activity levels.

10.   Focus on whole, nutrient-dense foods and prioritize quality over quantity.

Whole30 Diet:

Definition:

The Whole30 diet is a 30-day elimination diet designed to reset your body and identify potential food sensitivities. It involves removing certain food groups known to cause inflammation and digestive issues, such as sugar, grains, dairy, legumes, and processed foods, for 30 days. After the elimination period, foods are gradually reintroduced to identify which ones may be causing adverse reactions.

Ingredients:

- Protein Sources: Meat, poultry, fish, seafood, eggs.

- Vegetables: Leafy greens, cruciferous vegetables, peppers, squash, etc.

- Fruits: Berries, apples, oranges, bananas, etc.

- Healthy Fats: Avocado, olive oil, coconut oil, nuts, seeds.

- Herbs and Spices: Basil, oregano, garlic, turmeric, cinnamon, etc.

Instructions/How to Prepare:

1. Eliminate sugar, grains, dairy, legumes, and processed foods from your diet for 30 days.

2. Base meals around protein sources, including meat, poultry, fish, seafood, and eggs.

3. Include a variety of vegetables for essential vitamins, minerals, and fiber.

4. Incorporate fruits as snacks or to add natural sweetness to meals.

5. Use healthy fats like avocado, olive oil, and coconut oil for cooking and dressing.

6. Experiment with herbs and spices to enhance flavor without added sugars or artificial additives.

7. Be mindful of hidden sources of sugar and processed ingredients in condiments and packaged foods.

8. Read labels carefully and opt for whole, minimally processed foods.

9. Stay hydrated by drinking plenty of water throughout the day.

10. After the 30-day elimination period, reintroduce eliminated foods one at a time and monitor for any adverse reactions or changes in symptoms.

Low-Glycemic Index Diet:

Definition:

The Low-Glycemic Index (GI) diet focuses on consuming foods that have a low glycemic index, which means they cause a slower and more gradual increase in blood sugar levels. This diet can help stabilize blood sugar, improve insulin sensitivity, and promote weight loss. Foods with a low GI typically include non-starchy vegetables, whole grains, lean proteins, and healthy fats.

Ingredients:

- Non-Starchy Vegetables: Leafy greens, broccoli, cauliflower, peppers, carrots, etc.

- Whole Grains: Quinoa, barley, bulgur, oats, brown rice, etc.

- Lean Proteins: Chicken breast, turkey, fish, tofu, tempeh, beans, lentils.

- Healthy Fats: Avocado, olive oil, nuts, seeds, fatty fish like salmon.

- Low-Glycemic Fruits (in moderation): Berries, apples, oranges, pears, etc.

- Herbs and Spices: Basil, oregano, garlic, turmeric, cinnamon, etc.

Instructions/How to Prepare:

1. Choose whole, minimally processed foods with a low glycemic index.

2. Base meals around non-starchy vegetables, whole grains, and lean proteins.

3. Incorporate healthy fats like avocado, olive oil, nuts, and seeds for satiety and flavor.

4. Limit high-glycemic foods such as refined grains, sugary snacks, and sweetened beverages.

5. Include low-glycemic fruits in moderation, focusing on berries, apples, and citrus fruits.

6. Be mindful of portion sizes and avoid overeating, even with low-GI foods.

7. Experiment with cooking methods such as steaming, roasting, and sautéing to enhance flavor and texture.

8. Eat balanced meals that combine protein, carbohydrates, and healthy fats to promote satiety and stabilize blood sugar levels.

9. Monitor blood sugar levels if necessary and adjust your diet accordingly.

10. Stay hydrated by drinking plenty of water throughout the day.

Low-Fat Diet:

Definition:

A low-fat diet is characterized by reducing the intake of dietary fats, particularly saturated fats and trans fats, to promote heart health, manage weight, and reduce the risk of certain chronic diseases such as cardiovascular disease. This diet typically involves limiting foods high in fat and choosing lean protein sources, whole grains, fruits, vegetables, and low-fat dairy products.

Ingredients:

- Lean Proteins: Skinless poultry, lean cuts of beef and pork, fish, tofu, tempeh, legumes.

- Whole Grains: Brown rice, quinoa, barley, whole wheat bread, oats, whole grain pasta.

- Fruits: Berries, apples, oranges, bananas, grapes, etc.

- Vegetables: Leafy greens, broccoli, carrots, bell peppers, tomatoes, etc.

- Low-Fat or Fat-Free Dairy: Skim milk, low-fat yogurt, reduced-fat cheese.

- Healthy Fats (in moderation): Avocado, nuts, seeds, olive oil.

Instructions/How to Prepare:

1. Choose lean protein sources such as poultry, fish, tofu, and legumes instead of high-fat meats.

2. Opt for whole grains like brown rice, quinoa, and whole wheat bread over refined grains.

3. Include a variety of fruits and vegetables in your meals and snacks for added vitamins, minerals, and fiber.

4. Select low-fat or fat-free dairy products to reduce saturated fat intake.

5. Limit added fats and oils, and use healthier cooking methods such as baking, grilling, steaming, or boiling.

6. Be mindful of portion sizes to avoid overconsumption of calories, even with low-fat foods.

7. Read food labels to identify hidden sources of fat and choose lower-fat options when available.

8. Incorporate healthy fats like avocado, nuts, and olive oil in moderation for flavor and satiety.

9. Stay hydrated by drinking plenty of water throughout the day.

10. Focus on overall dietary patterns rather than just reducing fat intake, and aim for a balanced diet that includes a variety of nutrient-dense foods.

High-Fiber Diet:

Definition:

A high-fiber diet focuses on increasing the intake of dietary fiber, which offers numerous health benefits such as improving digestion, promoting satiety, stabilizing blood sugar levels, and reducing the risk of chronic diseases such as heart disease, diabetes, and certain cancers. This diet emphasizes whole, unprocessed foods rich in fiber, including fruits, vegetables, whole grains, legumes, nuts, and seeds.

Ingredients:

- Whole Grains: Oats, barley, quinoa, brown rice, whole wheat bread, whole grain pasta.

- Fruits: Berries, apples, oranges, pears, bananas, avocados, etc.

- Vegetables: Leafy greens, broccoli, carrots, Brussels sprouts, sweet potatoes, etc.

- Legumes: Lentils, chickpeas, black beans, kidney beans, peas, etc.

- Nuts and Seeds: Almonds, chia seeds, flaxseeds, pumpkin seeds, sunflower seeds, etc.

- Healthy Fats: Avocado, nuts, seeds, olive oil, flaxseed oil.

Instructions/How to Prepare:

1. Incorporate a variety of whole grains, fruits, vegetables, legumes, nuts, and seeds into your meals and snacks.

2. Choose whole fruits and vegetables over fruit juices and refined grains to maximize fiber intake.

3. Include high-fiber foods such as beans, lentils, and chickpeas in soups, salads, and main dishes.

4. Replace refined grains with whole grains in recipes and meals, such as swapping white rice for brown rice or white bread for whole wheat bread.

5. Snack on raw vegetables with hummus or nut butter for a fiber-rich snack.

6. Add nuts, seeds, and avocado to salads, yogurt, or smoothies for added fiber and healthy fats.

7. Be sure to drink plenty of water throughout the day to help move fiber through the digestive tract and prevent constipation.

8. Gradually increase fiber intake to allow your digestive system to adjust and minimize discomfort.

9. Monitor portion sizes, especially with high-calorie fiber-rich foods like nuts and seeds.

10. Aim to include a variety of fiber sources in your diet to ensure you're getting a balance of soluble and insoluble fiber, which offer different health benefits.

Flexitarian Diet:

Definition:

The Flexitarian diet is a flexible approach to eating that emphasizes plant-based foods while allowing for occasional consumption of meat and other animal products. It encourages individuals to primarily eat fruits, vegetables, whole grains, legumes, nuts, and seeds, while minimizing intake of processed foods, sugar, and refined grains. The diet is flexible and adaptable, making it suitable for various lifestyles and preferences.

Ingredients:

- Plant-Based Foods: Fruits, vegetables, whole grains, legumes, nuts, seeds.

- Lean Proteins: Tofu, tempeh, beans, lentils, chickpeas, edamame.

- Healthy Fats: Avocado, nuts, seeds, olive oil.

- Dairy and Eggs (optional): Greek yogurt, eggs, low-fat cheese.

- Occasional Meat and Fish: Lean cuts of poultry, fish, seafood (optional).

Instructions/How to Prepare:

1. Base meals around plant-based foods such as fruits, vegetables, whole grains, legumes, nuts, and seeds.

2. Include a variety of colorful fruits and vegetables to ensure a diverse intake of nutrients.

3. Incorporate plant-based proteins like tofu, tempeh, beans, and lentils into meals and snacks.

4. Choose healthy fats like avocado, nuts, seeds, and olive oil for cooking and dressing.

5. Limit consumption of processed foods, refined grains, and added sugars.

6. Enjoy occasional servings of lean meats, poultry, or fish if desired, but prioritize plant-based meals.

7. Be mindful of portion sizes and listen to your body's hunger and fullness cues.

8. Experiment with plant-based cooking techniques and recipes to discover new flavors and textures.

9. Stay hydrated by drinking plenty of water throughout the day.

10. Focus on long-term sustainability and balance rather than strict adherence to rules, allowing for flexibility and enjoyment in your eating habits.

Ornish Diet:

Definition:

The Ornish diet, developed by Dr. Dean Ornish, is a low-fat, plant-based eating plan designed to prevent and reverse heart disease and promote overall health and well-being. It emphasizes whole, unprocessed foods such as fruits, vegetables, whole grains, legumes, and limited amounts of low-fat dairy and plant-based proteins. The diet also encourages regular exercise, stress management, and social support as part of a holistic approach to health.

Ingredients:

- Plant-Based Foods: Fruits, vegetables, whole grains, legumes, nuts, seeds.

- Low-Fat Dairy: Skim milk, low-fat yogurt, cottage cheese (in moderation).

- Lean Proteins: Tofu, tempeh, beans, lentils, chickpeas, edamame.

- Healthy Fats (in moderation): Avocado, nuts, seeds, olive oil.

- Occasional Fish (optional): Fatty fish like salmon, trout, sardines (in moderation).

Instructions/How to Prepare:

1. Base meals around plant-based foods such as fruits, vegetables, whole grains, legumes, nuts, and seeds.

2. Include a variety of colorful fruits and vegetables to ensure a diverse intake of nutrients.

3. Choose low-fat dairy products like skim milk, low-fat yogurt, and cottage cheese in moderation.

4. Incorporate plant-based proteins like tofu, tempeh, beans, and lentils into meals and snacks.

5. Limit consumption of added fats and oils, opting for healthier sources like avocado, nuts, seeds, and olive oil.

6. Minimize intake of animal products, particularly high-fat meats and full-fat dairy.

7. Focus on whole, unprocessed foods and avoid processed and refined foods.

8. Practice stress management techniques such as meditation, yoga, or deep breathing exercises.

9. Engage in regular physical activity, aiming for at least 30 minutes of moderate exercise most days of the week.

10. Cultivate a supportive social network and prioritize meaningful connections with friends and loved ones for overall well-being.

TLC Diet (Therapeutic Lifestyle Changes):

Definition:

The TLC diet is a heart-healthy eating plan designed to reduce cholesterol levels and lower the risk of heart disease. It emphasizes reducing intake of saturated fat and dietary cholesterol while focusing on consuming a variety of nutrient-rich foods, including fruits, vegetables, whole grains, lean proteins, and healthy fats. The diet also encourages regular physical activity and other lifestyle modifications to promote heart health.

Ingredients:

- Fruits: Berries, apples, oranges, bananas, grapes, etc.

- Vegetables: Leafy greens, broccoli, carrots, bell peppers, tomatoes, etc.

- Whole Grains: Oats, barley, quinoa, brown rice, whole wheat bread, whole grain pasta.

- Lean Proteins: Skinless poultry, fish, seafood, tofu, beans, lentils.

- Healthy Fats: Avocado, nuts, seeds, olive oil, fatty fish like salmon.

- Low-Fat or Fat-Free Dairy: Skim milk, low-fat yogurt, reduced-fat cheese.

- Herbs and Spices: Basil, oregano, garlic, turmeric, cinnamon, etc.

Instructions/How to Prepare:

1. Limit intake of saturated fats, trans fats, and dietary cholesterol by choosing lean proteins, low-fat dairy products, and healthy fats.

2. Focus on consuming a variety of colorful fruits and vegetables for essential vitamins, minerals, and antioxidants.

3. Choose whole grains over refined grains for added fiber and nutrients.

4. Incorporate lean proteins such as poultry, fish, tofu, beans, and lentils into meals and snacks.

5. Use healthy fats like avocado, nuts, seeds, and olive oil for cooking and dressing.

6. Limit consumption of processed foods, sugary snacks, and high-fat meats.

7. Be mindful of portion sizes to avoid overeating, especially with calorie-dense foods.

8. Read food labels to identify hidden sources of saturated and trans fats, sodium, and added sugars.

9. Stay hydrated by drinking plenty of water throughout the day.

10.   Engage in regular physical activity, aiming for at least 30 minutes of moderate exercise most days of the week to complement dietary changes and promote overall heart health.

FODMAP Diet (Fermentable Oligosaccharides, Disaccharides, Monosaccharides, and Polyols):

Definition:

The FODMAP diet is a therapeutic approach to managing symptoms of irritable bowel syndrome (IBS) and other gastrointestinal disorders. It involves temporarily reducing or eliminating certain types of carbohydrates that are poorly absorbed in the small intestine and can ferment in the colon, leading to gas, bloating, abdominal pain, and other digestive symptoms. The diet consists of three phases: elimination, reintroduction, and personalization.

Ingredients:

- Low-FODMAP Fruits: Berries, citrus fruits, bananas, grapes, kiwi, etc.

- Low-FODMAP Vegetables: Leafy greens, carrots, bell peppers, zucchini, potatoes, etc.

- Low-FODMAP Grains: Quinoa, rice (white and brown), oats (gluten-free), etc.

- Low-FODMAP Proteins: Chicken, turkey, fish, eggs, tofu, tempeh, firm tofu, etc.

- Low-FODMAP Dairy: Lactose-free milk, lactose-free yogurt, hard cheeses (e.g., cheddar), etc.

- Low-FODMAP Fats and Oils: Olive oil, coconut oil, butter (in moderation), etc.

- Herbs and Spices: Basil, oregano, ginger, turmeric, cinnamon, etc.

Instructions/How to Prepare:

1. Start with the elimination phase, during which high-FODMAP foods are eliminated from the diet for 2-6 weeks to reduce symptoms.

2. Base meals around low-FODMAP foods such as fruits, vegetables, grains, proteins, and fats that are well-tolerated.

3. Gradually reintroduce high-FODMAP foods one at a time in small portions to identify trigger foods and tolerance levels.

4. Keep a food and symptom diary to track reactions to specific foods and help identify patterns.

5. Personalize the diet by incorporating a variety of low-FODMAP foods that are well-tolerated and avoiding or limiting high-FODMAP foods that trigger symptoms.

6. Be mindful of portion sizes and avoid overeating, as consuming large quantities of even low-FODMAP foods can exacerbate symptoms.

7. Consider working with a registered dietitian experienced in the FODMAP diet to ensure proper implementation and guidance throughout the process.

8. Stay hydrated by drinking plenty of water throughout the day to support digestive health.

9. Experiment with cooking methods and recipes to add flavor and variety to meals while adhering to the low-FODMAP guidelines.

10. Monitor symptoms regularly and adjust your diet as needed to manage symptoms effectively and improve overall quality of life.

Pescatarian Diet:

Definition:

The pescatarian diet is a plant-based eating pattern that includes fish and seafood but excludes other animal meats such as poultry, beef, and pork. It's a flexible approach to eating that emphasizes plant foods such as fruits, vegetables, whole grains, legumes, nuts, and seeds, while also incorporating fish and seafood for protein and essential nutrients like omega-3 fatty acids.

Ingredients:

- Fish and Seafood: Salmon, trout, tuna, mackerel, shrimp, scallops, etc.

- Plant-Based Foods: Fruits, vegetables, whole grains, legumes, nuts, seeds.

- Dairy and Eggs: Milk, cheese, yogurt, eggs (optional, depending on individual preferences).

- Healthy Fats: Avocado, olive oil, nuts, seeds.

- Herbs and Spices: Basil, oregano, garlic, turmeric, ginger, etc.

Instructions/How to Prepare:

1. Base meals around plant-based foods such as fruits, vegetables, whole grains, legumes, nuts, and seeds.

2. Incorporate fish and seafood into meals as the primary source of protein.

3. Choose fatty fish like salmon, mackerel, and trout for their omega-3 fatty acids.

4. Include dairy products and eggs if desired and tolerated, as they provide additional protein and nutrients.

5. Use healthy fats like avocado, olive oil, nuts, and seeds for cooking and dressing.

6. Experiment with a variety of cooking methods, such as grilling, baking, steaming, and sautéing, to enhance flavor and texture.

7. Be mindful of portion sizes and aim for balanced meals that include a variety of food groups.

8. Opt for whole, minimally processed foods and limit intake of processed and refined foods.

9. Stay hydrated by drinking plenty of water throughout the day.

10. Consider supplementing with vitamin B12 and vitamin D if fish and seafood are the primary sources of these nutrients in the diet.

Nordic Diet:

Definition:

The Nordic diet is a traditional eating pattern inspired by the cuisines of countries in the Nordic region, such as Denmark, Finland, Iceland, Norway, and Sweden. It emphasizes seasonal, locally sourced foods that are typical of the region, including fish, seafood, whole grains, berries, root vegetables, legumes, and rapeseed oil. The diet is characterized by its high fiber, low glycemic index, and focus on quality ingredients.

Ingredients:

- Fish and Seafood: Salmon, herring, mackerel, cod, trout, shrimp, etc.

- Whole Grains: Rye bread, barley, oats, quinoa, whole grain pasta.

- Berries: Blueberries, lingonberries, raspberries, cloudberries, etc.

- Vegetables: Root vegetables (e.g., carrots, potatoes, beets), leafy greens, cabbage, onions, etc.

- Legumes: Beans, lentils, peas.

- Rapeseed Oil: Used for cooking and dressing.

- Dairy: Milk, cheese, yogurt (in moderation).

- Herbs and Spices: Dill, parsley, thyme, juniper berries, etc.

Instructions/How to Prepare:

1. Base meals around seasonal, locally sourced foods typical of the Nordic region.

2. Include fish and seafood as the primary sources of protein, aiming for 2-3 servings per week.

3. Incorporate whole grains such as rye bread, barley, oats, and quinoa into meals for fiber and nutrients.

4. Enjoy a variety of berries, which are rich in antioxidants and vitamins.

5. Include plenty of vegetables, particularly root vegetables, leafy greens, and cabbage.

6. Incorporate legumes like beans, lentils, and peas into soups, stews, and salads for plant-based protein and fiber.

7. Use rapeseed oil for cooking and dressing, as it's a traditional oil in Nordic cuisine and rich in omega-3 fatty acids.

8. Include dairy products like milk, cheese, and yogurt in moderation, opting for low-fat or fermented varieties.

9. Flavor dishes with traditional Nordic herbs and spices like dill, parsley, thyme, and juniper berries.

10. Be mindful of portion sizes and aim for balanced meals that include a variety of food groups, focusing on quality ingredients and seasonal produce.

Asian Diet:

Definition:

The Asian diet refers to the traditional eating patterns of countries in the Asian continent, which vary greatly depending on the region and cultural influences. However, some common characteristics include a high consumption of plant-based foods such as fruits, vegetables, whole grains, legumes, and nuts; moderate intake of lean proteins such as fish, poultry, tofu, and eggs; and limited consumption of red meat and processed foods. The Asian diet is known for its emphasis on balance, variety, and moderation, as well as the inclusion of herbs, spices, and fermented foods for flavor and health benefits.

Ingredients:

- Rice: White rice, brown rice, jasmine rice, basmati rice, etc.

- Vegetables: Leafy greens, bok choy, broccoli, cabbage, carrots, onions, garlic, etc.

- Seafood: Fish, shrimp, crab, squid, mussels, etc.

- Poultry: Chicken, duck, turkey (in moderation).

- Tofu and Soy Products: Tofu, tempeh, edamame, soy milk, etc.

- Fruits: Mangoes, papayas, lychees, durian, bananas, etc.

- Nuts and Seeds: Peanuts, cashews, almonds, sesame seeds, etc.

- Herbs and Spices: Ginger, garlic, turmeric, coriander, cumin, chili peppers, etc.

- Fermented Foods: Kimchi, miso, soy sauce, fermented tofu, pickled vegetables, etc.

Instructions/How to Prepare:

1. Base meals around rice, noodles, or other staple grains, which serve as the foundation of many Asian dishes.

2. Include a variety of colorful vegetables in meals for added vitamins, minerals, and fiber.

3. Incorporate seafood, poultry, tofu, or soy products as sources of protein, aiming for a balance between plant-based and animal-based proteins.

4. Use herbs, spices, and aromatics like ginger, garlic, turmeric, and chili peppers to add flavor to dishes without relying on added fats or sodium.

5. Opt for cooking methods such as stir-frying, steaming, boiling, and grilling to retain nutrients and minimize added fats.

6. Include fermented foods like kimchi, miso, and soy sauce for their probiotic and digestive health benefits.

7. Enjoy fruits and nuts as snacks or dessert options, incorporating them into meals for added sweetness and crunch.

8. Be mindful of portion sizes and avoid overeating, focusing on listening to your body's hunger and fullness cues.

9. Stay hydrated by drinking plenty of water, green tea, or herbal teas throughout the day.

10.   Embrace the cultural diversity and culinary traditions of Asian cuisine by exploring recipes and ingredients from different regions.

Traditional Indian Diet:

Definition:

The traditional Indian diet is rooted in centuries-old culinary traditions and cultural practices, with a focus on balance, variety, and Ayurvedic principles of holistic health and wellness. It emphasizes plant-based foods such as whole grains, lentils, vegetables, fruits, nuts, and seeds, while also incorporating dairy products, lean proteins, and spices for flavor and medicinal purposes. The Indian diet is known for its use of aromatic spices, herbs, and cooking techniques that enhance both taste and nutritional value.

Ingredients:

- Whole Grains: Basmati rice, brown rice, wheat, millet, barley, quinoa, etc.

- Lentils and Legumes: Red lentils, chickpeas, black beans, mung beans, pigeon peas, etc.

- Vegetables: Spinach, potatoes, cauliflower, eggplant, okra, tomatoes, etc.

- Dairy Products: Milk, yogurt, paneer (Indian cheese), ghee (clarified butter), etc.

- Spices and Herbs: Turmeric, cumin, coriander, cardamom, cinnamon, cloves, ginger, garlic, etc.

- Fruits: Mangoes, bananas, apples, papayas, oranges, guavas, etc.

- Nuts and Seeds: Almonds, cashews, pistachios, peanuts, sesame seeds, etc.

- Lean Proteins: Chicken, fish, eggs (in moderation), tofu (less traditional), etc.

Instructions/How to Prepare:

1. Base meals around whole grains, lentils, and vegetables, which form the foundation of many traditional Indian dishes.

2. Incorporate a variety of lentils and legumes into meals for plant-based protein, fiber, and essential nutrients.

3. Use a wide array of spices and herbs to add flavor to dishes, such as turmeric, cumin, coriander, and ginger, which also offer medicinal properties.

4. Include dairy products like yogurt, paneer, and ghee for added calcium, protein, and healthy fats.

5. Opt for cooking methods such as sautéing, simmering, and pressure cooking to retain nutrients and enhance flavors.

6. Enjoy fruits as snacks or desserts, incorporating them into meals for natural sweetness and additional nutrients.

7. Include nuts and seeds in dishes or as snacks for added texture, flavor, and healthy fats.

8. Be mindful of portion sizes and avoid overeating, focusing on balanced meals that include a variety of food groups.

9. Stay hydrated by drinking water, herbal teas, or buttermilk throughout the day.

10. Embrace the cultural heritage and culinary traditions of Indian cuisine by exploring regional recipes and cooking techniques.

Low-Calorie Diet:

Definition:

A low-calorie diet is characterized by reducing daily calorie intake to create a calorie deficit, which can lead to weight loss. The focus is on consuming nutrient-dense foods that are lower in calories but still provide essential nutrients, such as vitamins, minerals, and fiber. This diet typically involves portion control, meal planning, and making healthier food choices to achieve and maintain a healthy weight.

Ingredients:

- Lean Proteins: Skinless poultry, fish, seafood, tofu, tempeh, legumes.

- Non-Starchy Vegetables: Leafy greens, broccoli, cauliflower, bell peppers, zucchini, etc.

- Whole Grains (in moderation): Quinoa, brown rice, whole wheat bread, oats, barley.

- Fruits (in moderation): Berries, apples, oranges, bananas, melons, etc.

- Healthy Fats (in moderation): Avocado, nuts, seeds, olive oil.

- Low-Calorie Flavor Enhancers: Herbs, spices, vinegar, lemon juice, mustard, hot sauce.

Instructions/How to Prepare:

1. Calculate your daily calorie needs based on your age, gender, weight, height, and activity level.

2. Set a calorie goal that creates a calorie deficit for weight loss, typically 500 to 1000 calories less than your maintenance calories.

3. Plan meals that include lean proteins, non-starchy vegetables, whole grains (in moderation), fruits (in moderation), and healthy fats (in moderation).

4. Incorporate low-calorie flavor enhancers such as herbs, spices, vinegar, lemon juice, mustard, and hot sauce to add flavor without adding extra calories.

5. Be mindful of portion sizes and avoid oversized servings, using smaller plates and utensils if necessary.

6. Focus on filling half of your plate with non-starchy vegetables to add volume and fiber to meals while keeping calories low.

7. Choose lean protein sources like skinless poultry, fish, tofu, and legumes to help satisfy hunger and maintain muscle mass.

8. Include whole grains and fruits in moderation for added nutrients and fiber, but be cautious of portion sizes to manage calorie intake.

9. Incorporate healthy fats like avocado, nuts, seeds, and olive oil into meals to promote satiety and provide essential fatty acids.

10.	Stay hydrated by drinking plenty of water throughout the day, as thirst can sometimes be mistaken for hunger.

Gluten-Free Diet:

Definition:

A gluten-free diet involves eliminating foods that contain gluten, a protein found in wheat, barley, rye, and their derivatives. This diet is essential for individuals with celiac disease, an autoimmune disorder triggered by gluten, as well as those with non-celiac gluten sensitivity or wheat allergy. The gluten-free diet focuses on naturally gluten-free foods and gluten-free alternatives to grains containing gluten.

Ingredients:

- Naturally Gluten-Free Foods: Fruits, vegetables, nuts, seeds, legumes, meats, fish, seafood, eggs, dairy products.

- Gluten-Free Grains and Flours: Rice, quinoa, corn, millet, buckwheat, sorghum, amaranth, teff, gluten-free oats, almond flour, coconut flour, chickpea flour, etc.

- Gluten-Free Condiments and Flavorings: Tamari (gluten-free soy sauce), mustard, vinegar, herbs, spices, etc.

- Gluten-Free Snacks and Treats: Popcorn, rice cakes, gluten-free crackers, gluten-free cookies, dark chocolate, etc.

Instructions/How to Prepare:

1. Educate yourself about sources of gluten and read food labels carefully to identify gluten-containing ingredients.

2. Base meals around naturally gluten-free foods such as fruits, vegetables, nuts, seeds, legumes, meats, fish, seafood, eggs, and dairy products.

3. Choose gluten-free grains and flours as alternatives to wheat, barley, and rye, including rice, quinoa, corn, millet, buckwheat, and gluten-free oats.

4. Use gluten-free condiments and flavorings like tamari (gluten-free soy sauce), mustard, vinegar, herbs, and spices to add flavor to meals.

5. Be cautious of cross-contamination by using separate cooking utensils, cutting boards, and kitchen equipment for gluten-free foods.

6. Explore gluten-free alternatives to favorite dishes and snacks, such as gluten-free pasta, bread, crackers, and baked goods.

7. Experiment with gluten-free cooking and baking techniques using alternative flours like almond flour, coconut flour, and chickpea flour.

8. Be aware of hidden sources of gluten in processed foods, sauces, dressings, and packaged snacks, and choose certified gluten-free products when possible.

9. Check with restaurants about their gluten-free options and food preparation practices when dining out.

10.   Consider working with a registered dietitian or healthcare professional knowledgeable about gluten-free diets to ensure nutritional adequacy and dietary compliance.

Anti-Inflammatory Diet:

Definition:

An anti-inflammatory diet focuses on reducing inflammation in the body by emphasizing foods that have been shown to have anti-inflammatory properties while limiting or avoiding those that may contribute to inflammation. Chronic inflammation is associated with various health conditions, including heart disease, diabetes, arthritis, and certain cancers. The anti-inflammatory diet typically includes a variety of whole, nutrient-rich foods such as fruits, vegetables, whole grains, healthy fats, and lean proteins, while minimizing processed foods, refined sugars, and unhealthy fats.

Ingredients:

- Fruits: Berries, cherries, oranges, pineapple, papaya, etc.

- Vegetables: Leafy greens, broccoli, Brussels sprouts, cauliflower, sweet potatoes, etc.

- Whole Grains: Quinoa, brown rice, oats, barley, bulgur, whole wheat pasta.

- Healthy Fats: Avocado, olive oil, nuts, seeds, fatty fish (salmon, mackerel, sardines).

- Lean Proteins: Skinless poultry, fish, seafood, tofu, tempeh, legumes, beans.

- Herbs and Spices: Turmeric, ginger, garlic, cinnamon, cumin, basil, oregano, etc.

Instructions/How to Prepare:

1. Base meals around whole, nutrient-rich foods such as fruits, vegetables, whole grains, healthy fats, and lean proteins.

2. Incorporate a variety of colorful fruits and vegetables into meals and snacks for their antioxidants and anti-inflammatory compounds.

3. Choose whole grains like quinoa, brown rice, and oats over refined grains for added fiber and nutrients.

4. Include healthy fats like avocado, olive oil, nuts, and seeds in moderation to reduce inflammation and support overall health.

5. Opt for lean protein sources such as fish, poultry, tofu, and legumes, which contain anti-inflammatory properties.

6. Flavor dishes with herbs and spices like turmeric, ginger, garlic, cinnamon, and cumin, which have been shown to have anti-inflammatory effects.

7. Minimize consumption of processed foods, refined sugars, and unhealthy fats, which can contribute to inflammation.

8. Be mindful of portion sizes and avoid overeating, focusing on listening to your body's hunger and fullness cues.

9. Stay hydrated by drinking plenty of water throughout the day, as dehydration can exacerbate inflammation.

10.   Aim for a balanced diet that includes a variety of nutrient-dense foods while reducing sources of inflammation, and consider consulting with a healthcare professional or registered dietitian for personalized guidance and support.

Raw Food Diet:

Definition:

The raw food diet is based on the belief that consuming foods in their natural, uncooked state provides maximum nutritional benefits and enzymes that are destroyed during cooking. This diet typically includes raw fruits, vegetables, nuts, seeds, sprouted grains, and legumes, as well as some raw or minimally processed dairy products, eggs, fish, and meat. The raw food diet is high in vitamins, minerals, fiber, and antioxidants, and proponents believe it can lead to improved digestion, increased energy, weight loss, and reduced risk of chronic diseases.

Ingredients:

- Raw Fruits: Berries, apples, oranges, bananas, mangoes, etc.

- Raw Vegetables: Leafy greens, carrots, cucumbers, bell peppers, tomatoes, etc.

- Nuts and Seeds: Almonds, walnuts, cashews, sunflower seeds, chia seeds, flaxseeds, etc.

- Sprouted Grains and Legumes: Sprouted quinoa, lentils, chickpeas, mung beans, etc.

- Raw Dairy and Eggs (if consumed): Raw milk, cheese, yogurt, eggs (in moderation).

- Raw or Minimally Processed Meat and Fish (if consumed): Sashimi, ceviche, carpaccio, etc.

- Cold-Pressed Oils: Olive oil, coconut oil, flaxseed oil, etc.

Instructions/How to Prepare:

1. Base meals around raw fruits, vegetables, nuts, seeds, sprouted grains, and legumes.

2. Incorporate a variety of colorful fruits and vegetables into meals and snacks for their vitamins, minerals, and antioxidants.

3. Include nuts and seeds for healthy fats, protein, and fiber, using them in salads, smoothies, or raw energy bars.

4. Experiment with sprouted grains and legumes, which are easier to digest and may have increased nutrient bioavailability.

5. Be cautious with raw dairy and eggs, choosing high-quality, pasteurized options to reduce the risk of foodborne illness.

6. If consuming raw meat or fish, ensure it is fresh, high-quality, and properly handled to minimize the risk of foodborne pathogens.

7. Use cold-pressed oils like olive oil, coconut oil, and flaxseed oil for dressing salads or adding flavor to dishes.

8. Be creative with food preparation techniques such as blending, juicing, dehydrating, and marinating to enhance flavor and texture.

9. Be mindful of food safety practices when handling raw foods, including washing produce thoroughly and storing perishable items properly.

10. Listen to your body and adjust the raw food diet to meet your individual nutritional needs, and consider consulting with a healthcare professional or registered dietitian for personalized guidance and support.

Specific Carbohydrate Diet (SCD):

Definition:

The Specific Carbohydrate Diet (SCD) is a dietary regimen designed to manage certain digestive disorders, particularly inflammatory bowel diseases (IBD) such as Crohn's disease, ulcerative colitis, and celiac disease. It aims to reduce inflammation and promote healing of the gastrointestinal tract by restricting certain carbohydrates that are thought to exacerbate symptoms. The diet focuses on consuming easily digestible, nutrient-rich foods that are low in carbohydrates and free of complex sugars and starches.

Ingredients:

- Fresh Fruits: Apples, bananas, berries, melons, etc.

- Non-Starchy Vegetables: Leafy greens, carrots, cucumbers, bell peppers, squash, etc.

- Lean Proteins: Chicken, turkey, fish, eggs, tofu, tempeh, and certain cuts of beef or pork.

- Healthy Fats: Olive oil, coconut oil, avocados, nuts, seeds.

- Fermented Foods (in moderation): Yogurt, kefir, sauerkraut, kimchi.

- Certain Legumes and Beans (in limited amounts): Lentils, black beans, navy beans.

- Homemade Broths and Soups: Chicken broth, bone broth, vegetable soup.

- Natural Sweeteners (in moderation): Honey, maple syrup.

Instructions/How to Prepare:

1. Eliminate complex carbohydrates such as grains, processed foods, and sugars from the diet.

2. Base meals around fresh fruits, non-starchy vegetables, lean proteins, and healthy fats.

3. Choose easily digestible proteins such as poultry, fish, eggs, tofu, and tempeh.

4. Incorporate healthy fats like olive oil, coconut oil, avocados, nuts, and seeds into meals for satiety and energy.

5. Include fermented foods like yogurt, kefir, sauerkraut, and kimchi in moderation to support gut health and digestion.

6. Experiment with homemade broths and soups made from scratch using nutrient-rich ingredients.

7. Be cautious with certain legumes and beans, as they may cause digestive discomfort in some individuals.

8. Use natural sweeteners like honey and maple syrup sparingly, as they are allowed in moderation on the SCD.

9. Avoid processed foods, artificial additives, and preservatives, opting for whole, unprocessed foods whenever possible.

10.   Monitor symptoms and adjust the diet as needed to manage digestive issues and promote overall well-being, and consider consulting with a healthcare professional or registered dietitian for personalized guidance and support.

CHAPTER 12
A 31-DAY MEAL PLAN

Week 1:

Day 1:

- Breakfast: Greek yogurt with sliced strawberries and a sprinkle of almonds.

- Lunch: Turkey and cheese roll-up with lettuce and mustard.

- Dinner: Baked salmon with roasted asparagus.

Day 2:

- Breakfast: Oatmeal with sliced bananas and a drizzle of honey.

- Lunch: Spinach salad with grilled chicken breast, cherry tomatoes, and balsamic vinaigrette.

- Dinner: Stir-fried tofu with mixed vegetables and brown rice.

Day 3:

- Breakfast: Scrambled eggs with spinach and feta cheese.

- Lunch: Quinoa salad with cucumbers, cherry tomatoes, and lemon-tahini dressing.

- Dinner: Grilled shrimp skewers with zucchini noodles.

Day 4:

- Breakfast: Whole grain toast with avocado and poached eggs.

- Lunch: Tuna salad with cucumber slices.

- Dinner: Baked chicken thighs with roasted Brussels sprouts.

Day 5:

- Breakfast: Cottage cheese with sliced peaches and a sprinkle of cinnamon.

- Lunch: Turkey and vegetable stir-fry.

- Dinner: Baked cod with lemon and herbs, served with steamed green beans.

Week 2:

Day 6:

- Breakfast: Smoothie with almond milk, spinach, and berries.

- Lunch: Turkey lettuce wraps with hummus.

- Dinner: Beef stir-fry with broccoli and cauliflower rice.

Day 7:

- Breakfast: Whole grain waffles with Greek yogurt and sliced strawberries.

- Lunch: Chicken Caesar salad.

- Dinner: Grilled salmon with roasted sweet potatoes.

Day 8:

- Breakfast: Scrambled eggs with tomatoes and cheese.

- Lunch: Turkey and cheese sandwich on whole grain bread.

- Dinner: Stir-fried tofu with mixed vegetables and quinoa.

Day 9:

- Breakfast: Yogurt with mixed berries and a sprinkle of nuts.

- Lunch: Spinach and feta stuffed chicken breast.

- Dinner: Baked tilapia with steamed asparagus.

Day 10:

- Breakfast: Chia seed pudding with almond milk and sliced almonds.

- Lunch: Turkey and avocado wrap with lettuce and tomato.

- Dinner: Beef chili with kidney beans and diced tomatoes.

Week 3:

Day 11:

- Breakfast: Smoothie bowl with mango, banana, and granola.

- Lunch: Chicken and vegetable kebabs with Greek salad.

- Dinner: Baked chicken breast with roasted cauliflower.

Day 12:

- Breakfast: Whole grain toast with almond butter and sliced apples.

- Lunch: Tuna salad with mixed greens and cucumber.

- Dinner: Grilled shrimp with quinoa and roasted Brussels sprouts.

Day 13:

- Breakfast: Greek yogurt with sliced strawberries and a drizzle of honey.

- Lunch: Turkey and cheese roll-up with lettuce and mustard.

- Dinner: Stir-fried tofu with bell peppers and snap peas.

Day 14:

- Breakfast: Scrambled eggs with spinach and mushrooms.

- Lunch: Caprese salad with tomatoes, mozzarella, and basil.

- Dinner: Baked salmon with steamed broccoli.

Day 15:

- Breakfast: Cottage cheese with pineapple chunks.

- Lunch: Turkey and vegetable stir-fry.

- Dinner: Beef stir-fry with broccoli and brown rice.

Week 4:

Day 16:

- Breakfast: Smoothie with almond milk, spinach, and berries.

- Lunch: Turkey lettuce wraps with hummus.

- Dinner: Grilled chicken breast with roasted sweet potatoes.

Day 17:

- Breakfast: Whole grain waffles with Greek yogurt and berries.

- Lunch: Chicken Caesar salad.

- Dinner: Baked cod with lemon and herbs, served with quinoa.

Day 18:

- Breakfast: Scrambled eggs with tomatoes and cheese.

- Lunch: Turkey and cheese sandwich on whole grain bread.

- Dinner: Stir-fried tofu with mixed vegetables and cauliflower rice.

Day 19:

- Breakfast: Yogurt with mixed berries and a sprinkle of nuts.

- Lunch: Spinach and feta stuffed chicken breast.

- Dinner: Baked tilapia with steamed asparagus.

Day 20:

- Breakfast: Chia seed pudding with almond milk and sliced almonds.

- Lunch: Turkey and avocado wrap with lettuce and tomato.

- Dinner: Beef chili with kidney beans and diced tomatoes.

Week 5:

Day 21:

- Breakfast: Smoothie bowl with mango, banana, and granola.

- Lunch: Chicken and vegetable kebabs with Greek salad.

- Dinner: Baked chicken breast with roasted cauliflower.

Day 22:

- Breakfast: Whole grain toast with almond butter and sliced apples.

- Lunch: Tuna salad with mixed greens and cucumber.

- Dinner: Grilled shrimp with quinoa and roasted Brussels sprouts.

Day 23:

- Breakfast: Greek yogurt with sliced strawberries and a drizzle of honey.

- Lunch: Turkey and cheese roll-up with lettuce and mustard.

- Dinner: Stir-fried tofu with bell peppers and snap peas.

Day 24:

- Breakfast: Scrambled eggs with spinach and mushrooms.

- Lunch: Caprese salad with tomatoes, mozzarella, and basil.

- Dinner: Baked salmon with steamed broccoli.

Day 25:

- Breakfast: Cottage cheese with pineapple chunks.

- Lunch: Turkey and vegetable stir-fry.

- Dinner: Beef stir-fry with broccoli and brown rice.

Week 6:

Day 26:

- Breakfast: Smoothie with almond milk, spinach, and berries.

- Lunch: Turkey lettuce wraps with hummus.

- Dinner: Grilled chicken breast with roasted sweet potatoes.

Day 27:

- Breakfast: Whole grain waffles with Greek yogurt and berries.

- Lunch: Chicken Caesar salad.

- Dinner: Baked cod with lemon and herbs, served with quinoa.

Day 28:

- Breakfast: Scrambled eggs with tomatoes and cheese.

- Lunch: Turkey and cheese sandwich on whole grain bread.

- Dinner: Stir-fried tofu with mixed vegetables and cauliflower rice.

Day 29:

- Breakfast: Yogurt with mixed berries and a sprinkle of nuts.

- Lunch: Spinach and feta stuffed chicken breast.

- Dinner: Baked tilapia with steamed asparagus.

Day 30:

- Breakfast: Chia seed pudding with almond milk and sliced almonds.

- Lunch: Turkey and avocado wrap with lettuce and tomato.

- Dinner: Beef chili with kidney beans and diced tomatoes.

Day 31:

- Breakfast: Smoothie bowl with mango, banana, and granola.

- Lunch: Chicken and vegetable kebabs with Greek salad.

- Dinner: Baked chicken breast with roasted cauliflower.

THE END